The undiscovered causes of Lower Back Pain 2020

The undiscovered causes of Lower Back Pain

Eliminate the main causes to avoid the symptoms

AUGUST 15, 2020
Dr. Adnan Mizher Samarmad
Atlantic International University

Copyright

Title book: The undiscovered causes of Lower Back Pain 2020
Author book: Adnan Mizher Samarmad

Email address: amizher@icloud.com

ISBN 978-0-578-79156-2

Acknowledgments

On this occasion, I would like to extend my heartfelt thanks to the University and all the staff for sustaining its success.

I would like to extend my sincere gratitude to the President of the Atlantic International University, Dr. Franklin Valcin, for his successful management of the university. He provides an ideal image and effectively contributes by encouraging students to grow and succeed.

I would also like to thank my Adviser and counselor, Dr. Edgar Colon Lancara, and my academic /educational tutor, Mrs. Diana Salazar, for their unlimited warm support. I would like to thank my brothers, sisters, friends, followers, fans, and our employees and clients who assisted with the completion of this work and brought it this scientific and practical stage.

A special thanks to Dr. Arnold Rueegg, and Prof. Dr. Urs Fueglistaller from Switzerland for their holy and unmatched support toward my Dynasom concept of treatment LBP using the 1st –LBE. The author would like to thank Enago (www.enago.com) for the English language review.

This work is dedicated to the souls of the martyrs of the October Revolution in Iraq 2019 because they sacrificed their lives for independence, and freedom.

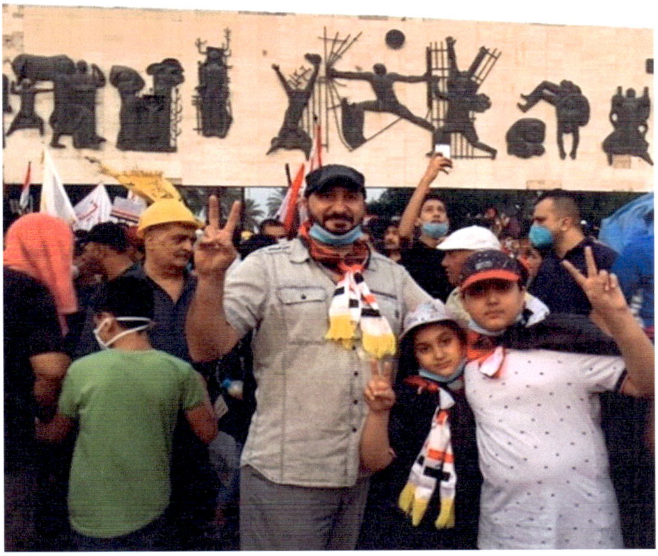

There are many people in Iraq who are looking for their healthy life and freedom. We should support them!

Abstract

To relieve lower back pain (LBP), one should identify the primary causes and eliminate them to prevent lumbovertebral syndrome that occurs in 80% of adults. In this thesis, I discuss and criticize the frequent use of spinal surgery and misuse of medication on the pretext of helping patients overcome LBP.

As an alternative, I invented a diagnostic and therapeutic concept called "Dynasom," involving non-surgical and non-pharmaceutical spinal care, based on the development of a first lower back extension (1st – LBE) anti-gravitation system, which can be used in spinal rehabilitation as a pre- and postoperative practices.

This system allows the diagnosis of the main causes of LBP, including dysbalance and weakness in the m. erector spinae. A leg length discrepancy (LLD) of 3–9 mm can be diagnosed during X-ray hips pelvis a.p. standing.

Through movement and dosage exertion on the 1st –LBE, I treated spinal disorders by improving the three-dimensional function of the spine. Consistent with spinal treatment, I compensate for LLD, at the site of existence, with orthopedic heel cushions, thereby eliminating one of the main causes of LBP in 70% of patients. This approach ensures spine functionality without medication or surgical intervention. To maintain the results, I recommend a maintenance program with daily regular movements, healthy and balanced nutrition, and cultivation of positive social communication. Finally, my aims match the third goal of UNESCO's 17 goals of sustainable development 2030: health and well-being.

Keywords: Undiscovered causes of Lower Back Pain, Spinal Instability, Leg Length Discrepancy and Spinal Disorders, LBP treatment without Medications, LBP treatment without Spinal Surgery, M. Erector Spinae System

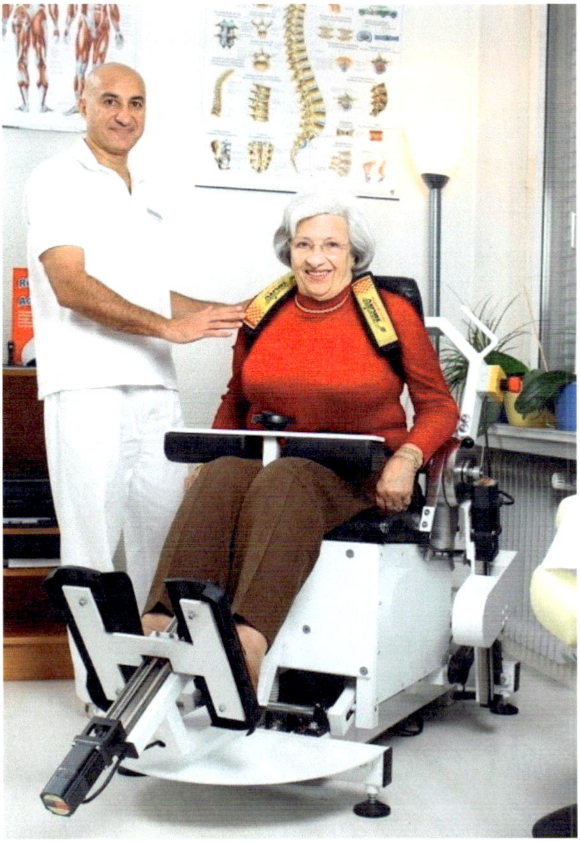

Dr. Adnan Mizher Samarmad treats his lower back patients with his self-developed device the 1st –LBE (Anti-gravitation System) in Switzerland, Germany and Iraq with a success rate of over 70% without medications or surgical interventions.

Table of contents

Chapter One

1. Introduction

Sitting for long periods, lack of exercise, stress, and monotonous activities— our modern way of life —brings with it a multitude of health risks.

In particular, our spine is exposed to great stresses and dangers. Currently, 60%–80% of adults are fighting pain in the back or musculoskeletal system that affects their well-being [1].

Back complaints reveal one of the most common types of suffering currently affecting the general population. Mechanical spine problems constitute the largest proportion of all acquired joint defects in the growth phase and adolescence. Scoliosis, spondylolisthesis, herniated discs, and spinal degeneration are the predominant spine conditions in modern society.

These directly affect the movement of the body, and cause spinal dysfunction, which leads to physical and mental health problems [2,3,4]. This negatively affects the well-being and economic situations of both the individual and society as a whole. LBP is the most common cause of a person's inability to work [5].

Overall, 600,000 jobs in Germany and Switzerland are lost every year owing to LBP, which also ranks highest as a cause of early retirement and in-patient rehabilitation. The annual cost of LBP in the USA is estimated to be 16– 20 billion dollars and disables 5.4 million Americans [1].

Research on innovative solutions for LBP is of great importance to the health and happiness of people in every society [6].

This thesis aimed to explore the main causes of LBP. Moreover, the study includes the link between the cause and onset of LBP and a method to overcome the painful symptoms naturally through movement with controlled exertion (Dynasom therapy concept) on the 1st – LBE (device).

Therefore, I primarily diagnosed the efficiency of the spinal muscles, m. erector spinae, and aimed to improve the support and balance to protect the spine and nerves, ultimately eliminating the causes of spinal distress that cause LBP.

Chapter two

2. Presentation of the problem

Lower back pain (LBP) is often considered a mechanical problem that develops when optimal functioning is reduced, causing the spine to become unstable.

This dysfunction plays an important role in LBP and its causes, acquired when the spine loses optimal movement during forward to backward, lateral left and right (L&R) or rotation movements. Causes include spinal instability that is mostly due to dysbalance and weakness of the muscular (m. erector spinae) and leg length discrepancy (LLD) [7].

Illnesses, sport injuries, accidents, and surgeries can also cause such problems; therefore, such events should be considered in the treatment.

In the normal growth stage, the spine is flexible and adapts to all of the conditions around it; the presence of abnormal growth factors clearly affect this adjustment. A LLD will cause a pelvic tilt [8], which is found in 70% of back patients [9]. Here the spine tries to adapt to the gravitational pull, possibly creating an uneven load on the intervertebral discs and vertebral joints, which causes an imbalance in muscle strength between the L&R sides, as well as between flexion and extension.

Consequently, the muscles cannot deliver their function optimally, the trunk cannot move easily, and pressure is placed on parts of the vertebrae, such as the intervertebral discs and joints.

These changes cause so-called incorrect posture, which leads to functional impairment of the spine. Thereby the statics and dynamics of the spine change and with it their biomechanics. The vertebrae no longer move properly toward one another, but rather they slide in the front, back, or to one side, disrupting the movement sequences.

This results in incorrect loading on the movement segments, which damages the movement elements including the intervertebral discs, joints, nerves, vertebrae, tendons, ligaments, and muscles [10]. Muscle imbalance between the right and left, or between flexion and extension, can occur through a wrong movement that is exercised continuously. Getting accustomed to a seated position can cause the same problem, and lead to the same imbalances and symptoms.

The consequences are imbalance and weakness of the inner back muscles (m. erector spinae), which has a negative effect on the spine components and complicates trunk movement, leading to malfunction and disturbance in the movement of the spine. The uneven pressure on the intervertebral discs and the ligaments, leads to disorder, wherein a sudden flare of LBP serves as a warning call; at the same time, the nerves become irritated and cause pain that radiates to one leg or both [10,11].

These small, uncontrolled movements between the vertebrae comprise spinal instability [10], which results in spinal dysfunction. From there, it can become a motion disorder, which in turn causes damage to the components of the movement and thus stimulates the pain to appear as an objector.

These are considered to be the cause of malfunctions in the spinal column. They develop undetected and cause malformations, thus laying the foundation for future spinal problems and LBP.

One of the most common causes of spinal instability is a difference in leg length, both functional and structural [11,12,13].

Weakness of the deep inner back muscles (m. erector spinae), along with an imbalance in the effort of the muscles between right and left plus flexion and extension, all of which play a major role in causing stiffness in the lower back.

The characteristics of the muscle fibers involved play an important role in the development of LBP or the protection of the spine from the problem [14].

Based on the principle that the body gives instructions before an injury occurs, I can assume that LBP gives instructions or warnings to the individual before it occurs. Such warnings may be represented by cramps or tiredness, or a slight tingling in the back.

An individual first needs to understand these signals in order to avoid the problem. Surely, an understanding of body attributes and the causes of pain is more valuable than applying a temporary treatment. It can also help the person overcome the problem and contribute to the success of the treatment, while avoiding a recurrence [15].

Indeed, some researchers have found that physical activities play an important role in maintaining health and promoting performance [16].

The WHO recommends physical activity to improve health. This can positively affect the heart, metabolic activity of the body, musculoskeletal system and cancer (breast and colon), and depression and preventive health. Individuals of all ages (5–17 years), (18–64 years), and >65 years should perform the following physical activities: Endurance training of intense (150 min) or average intensity (300 min) should be performed per week. Strength training for all muscles should be done 2–3 times a week.

For adults aged ≥65 years, the training program should be carried out with little intensity and no effort [17]. This line of reasoning has helped thought leaders and researchers in the field of LBP to consider that back pain appears when the defect is in the motion of the spine (dysfunction).

Accidents, sport injuries, diseases, and surgeries naturally play an important role in the appearance of LBP, particularly by changing the course of movement in order to adapt to the new situation.

However, the ability to recover and return to a normal state requires the person to first understand the problem and then eliminate the secondary effects, as well as to repair whatever is possible.

Therefore, a person's willpower plays an important role in healing. In athletes, for example, the will to succeed following an injury becomes clear because of the great motivation to return to the playing field [18].

At the same time, many researchers agree on the importance and role of muscles in overcoming the problems of movement of the human body, especially the spine, and often recommend non-pharmacological treatments [19].

The type of back muscle involvement (m. erector spine system) plays a major role in the identification of the pain character, and how to manage it.

Interestingly, there is a body of research on the results of magnetic resonance imaging showing people with bulges or protrusions of the spine but no pain in the back.

This phenomenon reveals that damage to discs does not have to cause LBP [20]. At the same time, I suspect that such conditions may represent a primitive stage in the development of a spinal problem. This is also evidence that these problems can exist for years before triggering pain alarms.

Broadly speaking, classical medicine does not always give importance to symptoms that do not fall within an established classification of disease. Such symptoms and suffering are considered normal, and chalked up to the person's psychological state [21,22]. I found it in >80% of my clients, many of whom go undiagnosed. That is why today we refer to LBP as a mechanical problem rather than a disease, and I feel certain that it will develop into an even bigger problem in the future.

Therefore, I categorized LBP into three levels (l, ll, and lll) based on the pain scale (0–3, 4–7, and 8–10) to facilitate the accurate diagnosis and serious approach to treatment of cases (this is a statement of my general approach to patients).

Chapter three

3. Goals and questions

Broadly, this research aimed to provide resources to therapists regarding the management of patients with LBP, facilitating diagnosis and correction of the causal factors, rather than simply treating the symptoms. It also explains the importance of the individual's understanding of his/her problem toward achieving success in getting rid of the pain.

The main objective of this work was to clarify the importance of diagnosing the causes of LBP and its treatment options. I developed the method described herein, which has been used in Switzerland since 2002, in Germany since 2011, and in Iraq since 2018.

This illustrates how to improve the function of the spine by moving against different levels of resistance to improve the toughness and balance of the back muscles. Secondly, on this device the torso moves with minimal axial pressure on the spine, which is achieved through balancing the upper body mass with the effect of gravitation, in other words through movement and controlled exertion therapy on the first lower back extension (1st –LBE).

This approach helps me to search for the link between the cause and the appearance of pain, and then overcome the painful symptoms in a natural way. I chose to rely mainly on diagnosing the efficiency of the m. erector spinae as a primary mover in spinal function, and aimed to improve the ability of these muscles to serve as an overall protector of the spine and nerves and thereby avoid the disorders that cause the pain. The therapeutic program included 12–18 treatment sessions twice a week for people were suffering from LBP for a period of > 12 weeks.

This research was oriented to answer the following questions - Which functional disorders on the spine need to be examined?

a) How do I search for the main causes of LBP?
b) How can I fix spinal dysfunction and treat the pain?
c) Why do I need 12–18 therapy sessions to overcome the pain and change the behavior of pain in patients with LBP?
d) How do I treat pain?
e) How can I find the differences between the types of fibers involved?
f) How can I make the results of successful therapy sustainable?

Chapter four

4. Overview of the literature

Types of LBP appear to range from mild to unexpectedly severe. If the pain is mild, it tends to disappear after some days and the person will often choose to not take any corrective action.

In such cases the situation will often repeat itself until the pain becomes keen and cannot be ignored [23]. The person may begin to think about this problem when the pain gets severe and effects movement, and ultimately determines their ability to perform activities of daily living or work. A person who finds themselves unable to perform their daily duties as easily as before [24] can lead to physical and psychological shock. This is often the moment that they decide to go to a doctor for help.

The first visit for a patient with LBP is typically the family doctor, whose first attempt is often to calm the patient and differentiate whether they are suffering from LBP due to factors at work or at home! The doctor may give the patient a break from work, and offer soothing medication for the pain. From this moment on, the marathon of LBP and its successions begins.

At this stage, the back patient is restless and afraid of the unknown, and so begins to look for solutions to relieve LBP that occurs regularly or unexpectedly. This level of thinking can lead patients down a long, difficult, and sometimes boring path. The suffering might end at the first physiotherapy station, or remain until the end of life.

In severe and critical cases, when the pain is strong, the doctor will typically continue to prescribe medication until the pain is relieved.

In the next sections, I describe the different stations that offer a solution for patients with LBP and analyze the positive and negative effects of each method.

4.1. Physiotherapy

Physiotherapy is typically the first stage of treatment for LBP. This method has proven its importance and development through scientific research as well as the development of technologies and various treatment methods [25], [26].

The most popular of these are massage, use of heat, manipulation, and infrared or ultraviolet radiation. They also include giving the injured party physical activity to exercise, either under their supervision or to be practiced later at home [27], [28].

At this stage, the therapist mainly depends on the diagnosis of the doctor who sent the patient. Yes, there may be some success in informing the patient, who now better understands the defect or damage to his back. Now he is ready to take responsibility for applying the instructed treatment at home to eliminate the problem.

The physiotherapist will also likely explain to the back patient how important it is to give the body enough time to relax, to ensure a healthy diet, and might attempt to motivate her to keep doing exercises to avoid a return of the problem. Overall these goals of physiotherapy aim to facilitate healthy life.

The weakness of this method lies in its generality. Generally, physiotherapists see many types of cases, not only LBP, and might lack sufficient information to diagnose the causes of the problem.

For this I recommend the further development of this specialist area toward the treatment of spinal column diseases. This can be achieved with scientific approaches such as radiology, muscle, and nerve physiology, and should also be accompanied by a focus on the biomechanics of the spine and information on how to deal with the possibilities for pain development in the m. erector spinae.

4.2. Sports Rehabilitation as a Supplement

The concept of sports rehabilitation has only recently been developed. This trend mainly relies on sports training methods and strengthening the back muscles especially as a way to overcome LBP [29].

Below are listed several examples for the delivery of sports rehabilitation.

1) David Back Klinik (DBK) has many years of experience in the conventional fitness area. DBK has started to focus on health, wellness, prevention, therapy, and the position physiotherapy market. The DBK spine concept is used in their own therapy centers and may also be carried out in traditional physiotherapy centers. Patient care is provided through the cooperation of different therapists.

2) Kieser training has its own centers. The idea of Kieser training is to counter back pain by strengthening the muscles [30], and is known all over Europe.

3) Health fitness training combines the health concept with fitness training, and also integrates wellness-oriented approaches. Like other health-oriented fitness centers, it focuses on preventive back training [38].

The concepts presented in competition analysis and similar analyses share main principle of building up the strength of the muscles in order to counteract LBP. This form of therapy has established itself as a classic concept.

Exercise is always good, but the concepts mentioned above are weak: there is no effective medical rehabilitation program, but only a focus on training the back muscles. In general, I and healthcare professionals know a large number of patients who are extremely strong but still experience pain. Strength is only a scientific aspect, nothing more. The exclusive primacy of strength is ideology.

4.3. Pain management

Local injections on the lumbar spine. In recent years, pain therapy has developed dramatically because patients are looking for a quick solution to their LBP.

The principle:

The local application of active ingredients, with both analgesic and anti-inflammatory properties, to certain parts of the movement segment has a direct influence on the pain in lumbar syndromes.

The reduction or elimination of pain results in decisive indications for the diagnosis and the therapeutic approach.

The injections are either remote from the segment, such as skin squeezing or trigger point infiltration, or close to the segment, such as paravertebral, epidural, intrathecal, perineural or facet infiltration.

The intradiscal injection has a special position. Depending on the intention, local anesthetics, steroids or both are used together for therapeutic local injection (TLI) on the lumbar spine.

For the diagnostic local injection (DLI) as a probatory injection, physiological saline is used first to provoke the typical pain, and in some cases contrast agents under X-ray control are used to determine the injection site.

If the pain is then switched off with a local anesthetic, it serves as a diagnostic, local anesthesia that leads to therapeutic local anesthesia.

When performing probatory local anesthesia to determine the starting point of pain, care must be taken that an anesthetic solution of only 1–2 cm^2 is used so that there is no scattering effect caused by anesthesia of the entire region.

The weakness of this method of treating LBP lies in its short-term effect; i.e. period of time, by affecting the pain. Likewise, after three doses, its effects disappear and the pain returns at the same level as before or even greater. more than it was!

Therefore, the patient continues to search for another alternative to relieve her LBP.

4.4. Osteopathy and chiropractic therapy

Osteopathy and chiropractic are the most popular methods for treating the motor system of the human body. They belong to the category of alternative medicine and mainly depend on the liberation of joints from restricted movement.

Their respective philosophies espouse the idea that human internal organs are involved in the disorder of the movement and support apparatus, and are considered scientifically controversial.

4.5. Traditional Chinese Medicine

Traditional Chinese Medicine (TCM) has long been established in conventional medicine, and its concepts have become more specialized in the health, wellness, and prevention sector, as well as in conventional and physical therapy treatment.

Outside of Asia, a TCM approach is primarily intended for customers who are looking for alternative medical solutions to their problems because they are not satisfied with conventional medicine.

TCM can be described as a small practice and has spread widely, with its spine therapy concept currently being used in some therapy centers.

TCM has experience in the area of back treatment with a focus on the health and therapy segment. The TCM concept delivers and installs various back therapy devices.

To ensure the desired therapeutic success, research efforts in TCM are working toward a quality management system. Patient care is provided through the cooperation of different therapists. At this stage, the biggest problem is when a patient has tried all of these approaches and still has pain. Here is when the side effects or even addiction to the drugs begins because the patient finds that medications are the only pain reliever.

During this stage, the patient may be tired or even exhausted by the pain and reviews of doctors and treatment centers. Losing her vitality and movement can impact her psychological state to the point that the apparent best solution becomes a surgery to get rid of the pain.

4.6. Spinal surgery

The subject of spinal surgery in medicine is controversial all over the world, namely because the financial interest of the clinics is greater than the effect of the supposedly scientific solution.

The following is a list of the most common spine operations: spine decompression, cleaning the spinal canal (laminectomy), herniated disc operations (discectomy), and spinal fusion (spondylodesis).

The intervertebral discs are partially removed by herniated disc operations, and artificially replaced in an intervertebral disc prosthesis operation.

However, the spine fusion operation blocks several movement segments, which eliminates the function of the intervertebral discs in the affected segments and puts more strain on other segments.

Suffering continues, leading patients to look for alternatives and something new: disappointment in the treatment of LBP by conventional medicine leads back patients to seek alternative treatments for their pain [30], [31].

This explains why many patients in every healthcare setting have not found a solution to their LBP, incur more problems after spine surgery, or suffer many adverse effects from pain medication.

In my opinion, these kinds of patients do not receive enough information about their problem to find the root cause and ideal solution through the classical medicine approach. This alone can make for a difficult life, as it has for my own father, sister, and brother.

That's why I consider this to be a gap in medicine, and one that has motivated me to do research, ask questions, and seek the right solutions.

After more than 20 years of work, it is a pleasure for me to present the efficacious results of my non-surgical, non-pharmaceutical method for spinal care of LBP.

Chapter five

5. Method: Necessity is the mother of invention

5.1. Development of the Dynasom concept

Throughout my life as an athlete, I have suffered many sports injuries. The most beautiful thing I learned from these experiences was how to get back on the sports field and with an even better level of performance than before the injury.

This feeling prompted me to invent a device that I named the 1st –LBE = Anti-Gravitation System as a way to solve the LBP problem. To analyze the movement of the spine and thereby uncover dysfunction, the apparatus measures every degree and newton in its three-dimensional motion.

This occurs by equating the human body's weight to gravity to reduce the vertical pressure that affects the spine between flexion and extension. I also use in this device different resistors to improve the balance and the toughness of the back muscles; up to a point, the m. erector spinae are responsible for protecting the spine by protecting the spinal cord and nerves.

My method is a statement of the diagnosis of motor dysfunction of the trunk (spine), the search for causes, and the treatment of the defect by overcoming the causes.

The first cause of the defect that occurs in the movement of the spine is an imbalance between the right and left internal muscles of the spine. This imbalance hinders the movement of the spine forward or backward (extension and flexion).

I also try to confirm this diagnosis through regular radiation: x-rays of the lumbosacral spine (anteroposterior [AP]/lateral standing), and the hips and pelvis (AP standing).

In the second stage, I look for any difference along the legs, while calculating its effect on the spinal function.

Important note:

A broad spectrum of knowledge along with specialized education in the fields of radiology, biomechanics, and muscle-nerve physiology of the spine are prerequisites for doctors and physical therapists who seek to implement my concept (Dynasom) and interpret their patients' progress with therapy using 1st –LBE technology (Fig.1). It is important to clearly understand the development of my diagnosis and treatment.

This doctoral thesis in health sciences by AIU will comprise some of the published results that are relevant to this project, as well as elements in my daily practice that are already in use. Based on the clinical use of my 1st –LBE device in Switzerland (2003–2010) and Germany (2011-2017), in the diagnoses of > 3,000 cases in Switzerland and Germany, and most recently in Iraq (2018–2020), I have published several papers, with full citations and abstracts where appropriate, as follows:

- Spinal Instability, Causes, Diagnostics, and Treatment. Original Study of 440

Patients. Author: Adnan Adeb Mizher. Publisher: Manuelle Medizin, Springer Medizin German. DOI 10.1007/s00337-012-0934-3/2012.

Abstract

Background. Acquired spinal instability is a biomechanical dysfunction and its development during or subsequent to the growth phase plays a major role in the progression of spinal diseases in adults.

Patients and methods. A total of 440 chronic and subacute low -back pain patients were evaluated. There were 179 males and 261 females ranging in age from 16 to 92 years (mean age male 48 years, female 53 years). The patient population was divided into two groups. (I) the first group consisted of 140 patients (32% of the population) who completed a total of nine sessions. (II) The second group consisted of the remaining 300 patients (68% of the population) who completed the whole program of 18 therapy sessions. The patients experienced spine symptoms on average for 8 months prior to the first evaluation. The two groups received the improvement of the three-dimensional lumbar spine functionality twice weekly.

Results. In group I a total of 56 patients (40%) experienced no improvement, however, 84 patients (60%) reported a significant improvement. In the second group 33 patients (11%) experienced no changes and 267 patients (89%) reported a significant improvement. For the second subgroup a maintenance program was continued with a further follow-up after 6–12 months.

Conclusions. Acquired spinal instability is a major contributing factor to the development of spinal diseases and it is therefore crucial to diagnose this early and to treat the dysbalance by improving the three-dimensional lumbar spine functionality. Optimal results in spine stabilization are achieved with an intensive program twice weekly for 18 sessions. This will assure that the spine is not only protected from early wear and tear but also from further pathological risks.

- Considerable Damage to Spine Caused by Small Leg Length

Discrepancy. Original Study of 210 Patients. Author: Adnan Adeb Mizher. Publisher: Manuelle Medizin, Springer Medizin, German. DOI 10.1007/s00337-016-0136-5/2016.

Abstract

Background. A LLD of 3– 9 mm causes mechanical and neuromuscular problems in the musculoskeletal system and particularly in the spine. This interferes the whole course of movement and is the main cause of degenerative changes of the spinal column, such as scoliosis, spondylolisthesis and disk herniation in adults.

Patients and methods. A total of 210 chronic and subacute low back pain patients (100 men and 110 women aged from 18 to 65 years) with leg length discrepancies of 39 mm were evaluated. The average duration of symptoms was 6 months. The patient population was divided into three groups: group 1 with 50 patients (24%) who received orthopedic heel cushions to adjust the LLD, group 2 with 50 patients (24%) who completed a total of 12 therapy sessions to improve the 3-dimensional lumbar spine function twice weekly and group 3 with110 patients (52%) who received heel cushions and completed the whole program of 12 therapy sessions. Therapy was carried out for 6 weeks in all groups.

Results. Evaluation of the data was carried out after 6 weeks with a follow-up after 6–12 months. In group (l) a total of 28 patients (56%) experienced no improvement but 22 patients (44%) reported a change for the worse. In group (ll) a total of 8 patients (16%) experienced no change and 42 patients (84%) reported a short-lived (1–2 days) improvement. In group (lll) a total of 15 patients (14%) experienced no change and 95 patients (86%) reported a significant improvement; therefore, a maintenance program was continued for group (lll) patients over a period of 6– 12 months.

Conclusions. A LLD of 3– 9 mm should be diagnosed early and appropriately treated. A correction using orthopedic heel cushions should help to improve the three-dimensional spinal function.

- Leg Length discrepancy promotes back pain. Manuelle Medizin 2017 DOI 10.1007/s00337-016-0194-8.

- **Back complaints can be resolved**. Manuelle Medizin 2017 DOI 10.1007/s00337- 016-0185-9.

- New Unpublished Study

Patients and Design: A retrospective analysis of patient records of 930 cases were I already used it in my practical work every day.

NEW: I diagnosed and treated in my Sporty Spine Center in Baghdad from August 2018 to August 2019. All of the patients 520 males and 410 females; age range, 15– 65 years; mean age for males, 45 years and for females, 50 years had suffered from LBP for > 12 weeks. The cases were divided into two groups: (I) 577 patients with a herniated disc causing local pain in the lower back and radiating pain, who comprised 62% of all cases; and (II) 353 patients with local pain in the lower back only (38% of all cases). Analysis of the two groups for spinal movement between flexion and extension showed an imbalance between the working of the spine muscles (m. erector spinae) located on the right and left sides. The two groups received the same balance correction in the spine (extension) with treatment effort (dosage exertion therapy program) applied over 12 sessions delivered twice weekly within 45 days.

Results. In group l, a total of 139 (24%) patients experienced no improvement, while 438 (76%) reported a significant improvement. In group II, 62 (18%) experienced no change and 291 (82%) reported a significant improvement. The evaluated data is a retrospective analysis of patient records.

Conclusions: We found that the causes of LBP in Iraq were similar to those in Switzerland and Germany, as were the success rates. These included weakness and imbalance in the inner back muscles, especially the m. erector spinae that cause spinal instability. LLD also played a major role in suffering from LBP in Iraq. These causes of LBP had not yet been diagnosed by medical facilities.

By improving the three-dimensional function of the spine (balance and toughness) with the 1st –LBE, and compensating for the LLD (where it exists), I am able to relieve 70%–80% of LBP in the spinal column of my patients.

For this reason, I consider LBP as a global problem, one that can be diagnosed and treated optimally with minimum medication or surgical intervention.

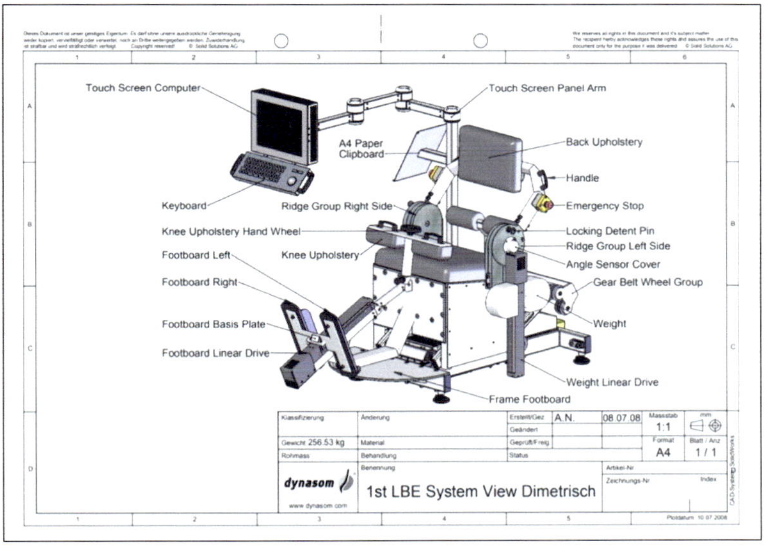

Fig. 1. The first Lower Back Extension (1st -LBE). Representing the first generation of lower back extension apparatus, this system works with an anti-gravitational technology that was developed by Adnan Adeb Mizher Al-Samarmad in Switzerland from 1999 to 2002, who has been practicing with it in Switzerland since 2003, in Germany since 2011, and in Iraq since 2018.

5.2. Basic considerations of the spine and gravity

5.2.1. Power is the source of motion

To move any particular mass requires force, and this force determines the speed or direction of the mass. Either the end of the stirring or any stop depends on the amount of strength gained by the body through its weight, through external influencing or through the power of stirring gained.

Furthermore, many external factors will hinder the movement and the external environment such as air and water or any other friction with the external surfaces, which acts as a resistance to impedes the movement.

However, in my opinion, that has no influence on the LBP development.

Gravity plays an essential role in the movement of all objects on the surface of the Earth's sphere. This is why many scientists study their dimensions and try to take advantage of them to serve humans, animals or nature.

My own work analyzing the effects of gravity on the movement of the human body has revealed its negative impact on the movement of the spine.

My overarching aim has been to assist with overcoming the gravity-associated difficulties that harm human health.

5.2.2. Spinal movement and gravity

I now know that the spine is directly affected by gravity. I have also proven that the consistency and balance of the spine depends mainly on the impact of gravitational attraction, and therefore I must study all possible ways to neutralize the collateral damage.

In my research, for example, I have shown that the difference in leg length attributable to gravity directly affects the coherence and balance of the spine.

Put simply, this means that our weight is a force in the down direction, which puts pressure on the joints, especially on the spine. Therefore, any movement will be influenced by gravity.

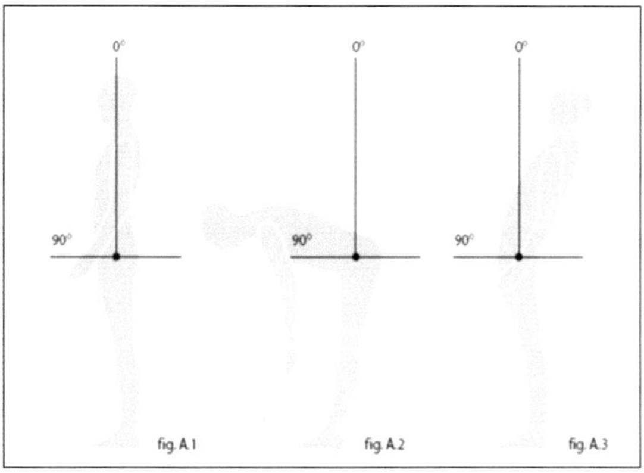

Fig. 2. The main movement of the lower spine in humans is to bend the trunk forward and back (flexion and extension); this movement is repeated >200 times a day.

The principle of unbalanced force is achieved between the weight of the trunk and the strength of muscles. Here the back muscles must provide sufficient strength to overcome the resistance, so that the process of moving the trunk toward the desired direction.

The position of the stand as shown in Fig. 2 (A. 1) is a movement of balance between the muscles of the abdomen and back to maintain the straight position of the body. Moving the trunk from the position in Fig. 2 (A. 2) to that in Fig. 2 (A. 1) will require the strength of the back muscles to overcome the weight of the trunk. This force gradually decreases as we get to a 0° position, and disappears completely in position Fig. 2 (A. 3); here the abdominal muscles operate in an unbalanced force to overcome the fall of the trunk toward the ground.

This effect does not require the back muscles in Fig. 2 (A. 3), which leads to weakness in the range of motion of this region, and over time the human body bends forward because it cannot lift the trunk weight. The inability of the back muscles to lift the weight of the trunk, i.e. a failure is to overcome gravity through muscle strength, leads to a defect in the spinal function maintaining the position of the trunk straight by moving as in Fig. 2 (A. 1).

The study of this principle of unbalanced force inspired me to work on developing strength in the deep back muscles of my patients moving between Fig. 2 (A.1) and Fig. 2 (A.3), to achieve a strong form between Fig. 2 (A.2) and (A.3) in order to reach Fig. (A.1) and maintain it.

By achieving this goal, we have been able to provide adequate protection of the spine in the daily movement between flexion and extension, lateral L&R, and rotation L&R, and thus overcome many common problems that result from the weakness of the spinal muscles in the development of the main function of the spine three-dimensional movement = extension in toughness + balance), namely herniated discs, spondylolisthesis, scoliosis, and degenerative diseases.

I was able to use ground gravity to weigh the trunk of the human body, turn it to generate a controlled resistance by which it developed the range of motion to overcome weakness in the deep muscles of the spine (m. erector spinae system), and thus transform the attractive ground from the negative to the positive.

My 1st –LBE also uses the ground gravity (unbalanced force) between the movement of the spine and the measured and regulated resistance to develop the muscles of the spine gradually.

The goal was to develop muscle strength to a certain extent (60% of the weight of the human body) to overcome the gravity of the ground and minimize the axial pressure on the spine (Figs. 3,4), which helps to reduce the injuries of the spine and maintain its effectiveness at providing the optimal position to protect the spinal cord and nerves from unwanted pressures (injuries).

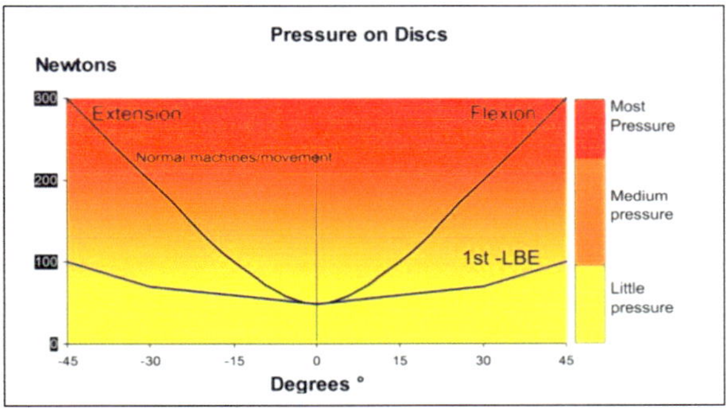

Fig. 3. The 1st-LBE minimizes the pressure on Discs by movement. This is how I made the difference

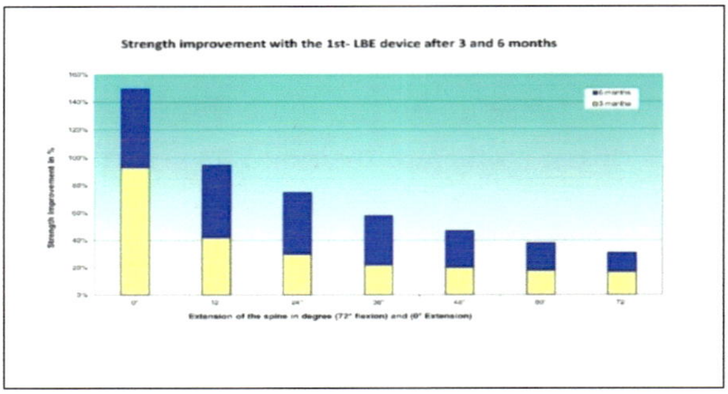

Fig. 4. Therapy effect (strength improvement) with the 1st -LBE after 3 and 6 months

Average isometric strength increase in each position after 3 and 6 months of treatment. The (expected) biggest increase was shown at 0° extensions. Here atrophy is usually most pronounced (Fig. 4).

However, based on practical experience, we have found that the pain in the lower back causes a restriction of movement that leads to an inability of the spine to ensure the desired three dimensional movement of the trunk.

Also, I found that the average person, not the athlete, had to improve the toughness and balance of the back muscles to a 45– 51° flexion and a 9–6° extension to ensure the necessary spinal function for daily requirements. The 1st –LBE uses the weight of the patient to create 20 levels of resistance, each accounting for 5% of the body weight.

In the beginning of my sports life at age of 17, I was suffering from severe pain in my left ankle. I had it checked by doctors of sports medicine, but none of them recognized the causes of my problem, so I used a tightly tied bandage until I finished competing in a championship event. Unfortunately, I continued to suffer from pain for another a week before it calmed down.

At an international championship at the age of 23, I had an injury to my right knee (inner ligaments with small torn cartilage). After my review by sports medical experts, they recommended that I have an operation to remove all of the cartilage because they didn't know the cause of the injury. At the end of my athletic career, an injury of the right pelvic joint caused me to stop participating in international championships.

During this time, I had pain in the lower back on the right side, accompanied by pain in the neck on the same side. This lumbago has recurred > 10 times over a 2-year period, and has troubled me with great pain lasting an entire week. In addition, no sports medicine expert has been able to identify the cause or provide a way to treat or prevent the problem from recurring.

Through scientific research and investigation into the causes of this suffering and painful experience, I found that the length of my right leg was 5 mm shorter than the left, which caused minimal functional scoliosis (spinal instability). That was the main reason for not only my LBP, but also all of the other sports injuries that had occurred during my sports life.

After diagnosing and treating thousands of cases in Switzerland, Germany, and most recently Iraq, for the past 20 years, I have found that many people suffer from these symptoms. Experts typically do not correctly identify nor explain the cause of their patients' pain.

For this reason, I recommended that all patients to look for the causes that have been mentioned in this thesis, discuss them with their hired experts, and take responsibility for themselves.

Indeed, this requires a certain amount of knowledge, which should be in the natural interest of the patient who truly desires to maintain good health.

The main concept of my method (Dynasom) includes the restoration and optimization of three-dimensional spinal function, which happens through improving the neuromuscular function of the m. erector spinae.

Conclusion: Gravitational force plays a vital role in human life and health. Understanding, its dimensions and its negative and positive effects will allow us to transform these influences and avoid the potential damage that results from it, turning it into usefulness.

For 20 years, I have analyzed the negative effects of gravity on the spine and used the base of the unbalanced forces to neutralize them. I aimed to create a muscle workout that would develop the spinal muscles so as to rid the spine of the mechanical problems that afflict it. It is my hope to further.

For these reasons, I recommend that all of our patients look for the causes that have been mentioned in this thesis, discuss them with their hired experts, and take responsibility for themselves to fix the problem.

Of course, this requires a certain amount of know-how, which should be in the natural interest of the patient who truly desires to maintain his health.

5.3. Diagnosis

The goal of my diagnosis is as follows:

Goal, the calculation of the pivot points, and the load distribution and limitation at each movement segment of the spine with compensation for the effect of gravitation (gravitational force).

The basic idea is that any vertebral shift can trigger pain or the basis of a pathological development such as scoliosis or spondylolisthesis, even if no pathological picture initially emerges, as a spinal instability.

5.3.1. Radiological diagnosis

In addition to the widely known spinal diagnoses, as part of the Dynasom concept, I examined the minimal translation of the lumbar vertebrae by analyzing the sacrum position and the alignment of the super-adjacent vertebral components.

Furthermore, I analyze the sacrum angle (SA) and the relation to TH 12 and to all sub-adjacent vertebrae (see Figs. 3 & 4) using AP and lateral x-rays. The structure and form of the individual vertebral bodies, including their configuration, influence the form and alignment of the entire lumbar spine.

This information is the foundation for a conclusive assessment of the individual biomechanics and functional deficits of the spine. Together with the patient's description of their ailment, my diagnosis is complete.

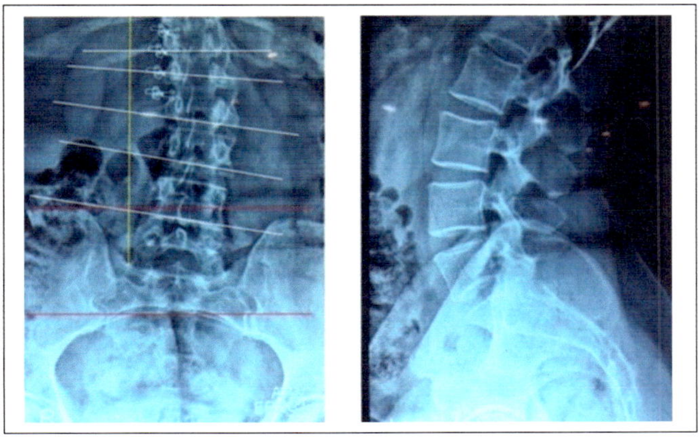

In Fig. 5.1., the AP view shows that the left translations of the vertebrae in the lower back cause unequal load distribution to the disks, which results in early wear and tear. Fig. 5.2, the lateral view, shows a dorsal translation of L5, L4, L3, and L2 of 2–3 mm each. These minimal Retrolisthesis caused by vertebral rotation thereby squash the intervertebral disks (axial and dorsal pressure with lateral and dorsal strain) and disrupt spinal movements.

5.3.2. Three-dimensional function diagnosis with the 1st–LBE

Using the 1st–LBE method, the dynamic functional examination takes place as part of the initial examination. I observe the patient's muscular balance and mobility stereotype (Figs. 6– 10).

The 1st–LBE apparatus shows the dysbalance between the left and right sides in the m. erector spinae caused by the scoliosis. This measurement allowed me to identify the cause of the disorder and treat it successfully.

It should be noted that 99 % of back patients have a dysbalance in the m. erector spinae system, independent of the pathological development, which can be observed as the cause of acquired physical spinal disorders.

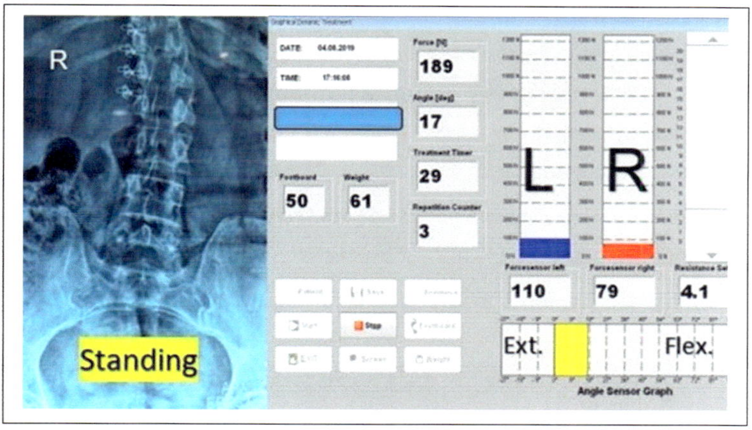

Fig. 6. A functional left convex scoliosis caused by LLD with an unequal load distribution along the intervertebral disks of a 39-year old patient (misalignment unequal load distribution = one-sided pressure).

5.3.3. Muscular function

The functional capacity and strength examination of all lumbar movement segments, a static muscular function and strength test of the m. erector spinae at preset angles of spinal extension, takes place on the 1st –LBE and is (repeated in the 3rd and 9th sessions of a course of therapy, and again at the end of a treatment series. The machine isolates the spinal muscles for testing purposes using fixations at the knees, hips, and shoulders. This allows for an exact measurement of muscle activity, including strength and balance (motoric nerve system) in all lumbar movement segments, which provides us with information on the biomechanics and construction of the spine as well as the individual strength capacity of the patient. The results of the static function and strength diagnosis are used to assess therapy progress and plan further spinal rehabilitation treatment.

The difference between the Dynasom concept and 1st–LBE device:

I developed the therapy concept and it includes diagnostic and therapeutic measures on the spine, which are carried out step by step. To implement the therapy concept, I needed certain movement and strength measurements (data), which I received from my self-developed 1st–LBE device.

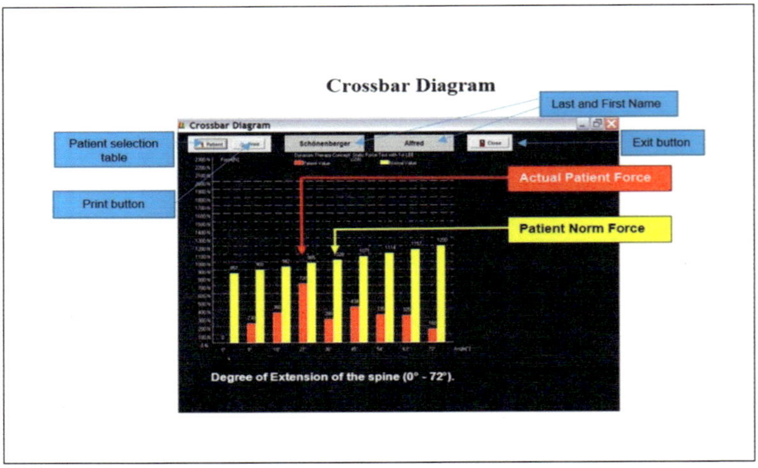

Fig. 7. The Crossbar Diagram displays the progress and improvement of the patient strength. The program first calculates the patient's norm values based on the patient weight. The patient's total force per angle tested is measured with the Static Force Test. The result of the Static Force Test helps evaluate the patient's progress and assist in the decision making for further therapy treatments. The diagram can be printed by selecting the print button, for safe keeping in the patients file.

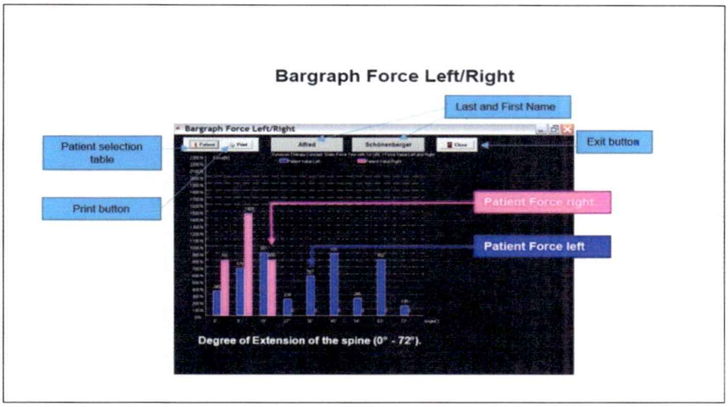

Fig. 8. The Bargraph Diagram reflects the static force value for the right and left side of the patient spine. This diagram displays the progress and improvement of the patient's strength and helps to evaluate their needs and further treatment requirements. The diagram can be printed to further document the patient's health history.

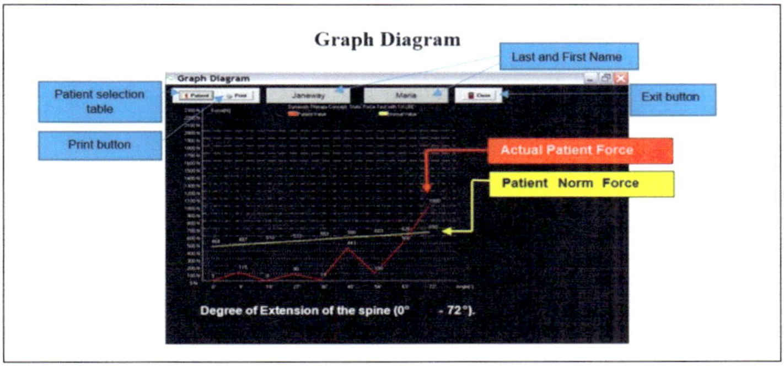

Fig. 9. The Graph Diagram displays progress and improvement in strength. This diagram enables the approximation of the force results in angles that are not measured with the Static Force Test, providing an alternative illustration of patient progress. The program calculates the patient's norm values based on body weight. The patient total force value is measured with the Static Force Test during the therapy session, and helps to evaluate the patient's needs and further treatment requirements. The diagram can be printed to further document the patient's health history

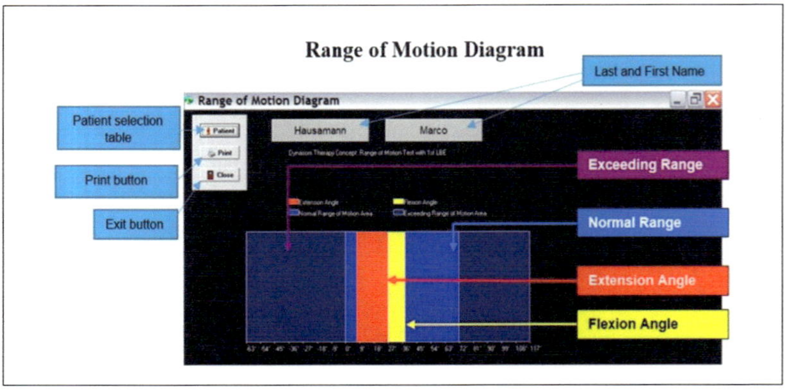

Fig. 10. The Range of Motion Diagram describes the patient's range of motion area in detail. This diagram visualizes the restrictions of the patient's extension or flexion range, can display improvements in range of motion, and can be printed to further document the patient's health history.

5.4. Lumbar spine therapy

The primary aim of my therapy method, Dynasom, is to examine the individual to determine the exact cause of the LBP. I then inform and guide her as to how to eliminate the causes of her unique problem.

This approach to eliminate pain can be realized by balanced movement and controlled exertion therapy to improve the toughness of the m. erector spinae.

I have consistently achieved these results in 80% of patients in Switzerland, Germany, and Iraq. Theoretically, this could be successfully applied to 70– 80% of spinal patients everywhere without medication or surgical intervention.

My approach to therapy is an active treatment that I have coined Dosage Exertion Therapy (DET), and is adapted to each patient based on their diagnosis (Fig. 11).

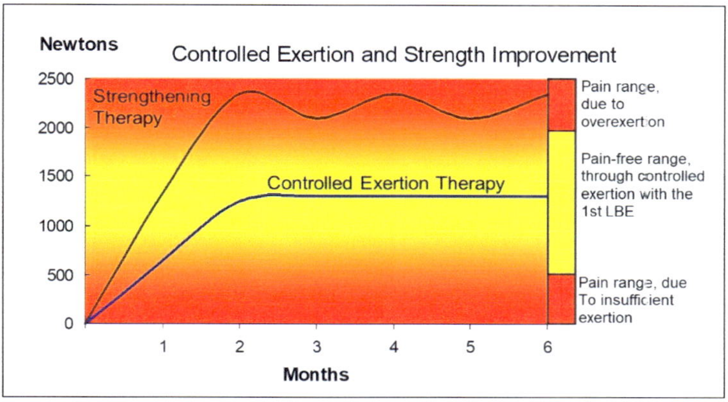

Fig. 11. The Dynasom Dosage Exertion Therapy with 1st -LBE

In accordance with the spine's main function, this active therapy consists of repeated extension of the over-stretched muscle fibers (weak side) of the lumbar spine (motion with dosage exertion) and depending on the established diagnosis, is combined with the lateral function, lateral flexion or rotation of the spine.

The aim is to alleviate the shortened muscles (strong side) to provide a dynamic correction that leads to an improvement in the spine's three-dimensional functional capacity. This is the main goal of Dynasom Dosage Exertion Therapy (Fig. 11), to improve muscle coordination (balance and toughness) by regulating the nerve impulses, which guarantees optimal spinal function.

To summarize, the functional goals of spinal rehabilitation according to muscular function in the Dynasom therapy concept are as follows:

1) even out muscular deficits (dysbalance and muscular atrophy)
2) re-establish joint stability
3) re-establish the physiological joint positions (according to the individual spinal construction) The dosage strength improvement

is targeted and efficient, and the muscles gain neuromuscular functionality as well as optimal (intermuscular) coordination.

Each therapy session lasted 20–30 min and included two therapy series. In each series there are 20– 30 repetitions within 150 s (submaximal = anaerobic load) with a break of 1–2 minutes between the series. The physical therapy was performed twice a week for 6 weeks.

Patients completed the pain questionnaire before and 6 weeks after therapy (12 sessions; conclusion of therapy). The follow-up pain questionnaire was not completed until 6–12 months after therapy completion.

5.4.1. Diagnostic measures during the course of therapy

As therapy progresses, it is important to reconfirm the diagnosis and adjust the treatment plan as necessary. A patient's subjective information (i.e. perceived reactions) is central to further treatment progression.

Individual strength capacity depends on the patient's diagnosis, symptoms, constitution, and condition. Specific muscular differences, such as muscular deficit pain or reduced regenerative ability, can only be diagnosed through an individualized strength improvement treatment of the spinal muscles.

My most important duties are not only to identify the patient's type of back muscle fibers, but also to investigate the reactions and limitations of movement to examine the appropriate load for each patient to achieve optimal spinal stability.

The muscle fibers of the m. erector spinae must be closely monitored, analyzed, and documented.

The muscle fibers are predetermined by hereditary systems. A distinction is made between the thinner, dark-colored, so-called red muscle fibers, and the thicker, pale colored, so-called white fibers. The color difference is due to the content of red muscle pigment, myoglobin.

The intermediate muscle fibers lie between these two fiber types. The white muscle fibers are characterized by a high contraction and exhaustion speed, and are also referred to as fast- twitch fibers. In contrast, the red muscle fibers are characterized as slow- twitch fibers.

5.4.2. Distribution of fiber types

a) Approximately 10% of patients are fast-twitch fiber dominant; inroad > 30%
b) Approximately 10% of patients are slow-twitch fiber dominant; inroad < 10%
c) Approximately 80% of patients are balanced type; inroad 10%–30%

Definitions: inroad = loss of power as a result of dynamic resistance.

These fiber type characteristics affect my treatment, in particular by indicating the resistance and the time.

a) Fast-twitch patients should be treated for short times (60–90 s) with more resistance (60%–80% of the patient's body weight).
b) Slow-twitch, should be treated for longer times (130–150 s) with less resistance (40%– 60% of body weight).
c) Mixed fast- and slow-twitch patients, should be treated with an average time (110–130 s) and average resistance (60%–80% of body weight).

Older-age patients (65 and over) should be treated for up to 120 seconds with a resistance of 50%–60% of body weight.

Clinical importance of muscle fibers and leg length discrepancy in this project.

The strain on the m. erector spinae system causes paravertebral - burning pain after 50–60 seconds in fast twitch fibers, which immediately disappears when the load is interrupted.

This physiological pain response arises from the muscle tension caused by the white muscle fibers. However, this muscle reaction can lead to pathological development [14].

In response to pain relief, there is a weakening of the deep back muscles. This places unnecessary or uneven stress on other spine structures, such as the vertebral bodies, intervertebral discs, joints and ligaments, and causes problems including lumbar spine syndrome. The error described below often occurs in conservative spine treatment.

A LLD is discovered and compensated with a heel cushion without taking into account the function and stability of the spine. This results in static and dynamic positions, instabilities in different movement segments, and new incorrect postures as well as incorrect loads on the spine.

The consequences are unexpected complaints that unsettle the patient, and confidence in the treatment and healthcare professional is lost. Therefore, the stability of the spine should be the initial focus of treatment, followed by efforts to compensate for the LLD. As part of the interim control and treatment success, the entire difference must be compensated.

5.4.3. Effects of the therapy

The Dynasom therapy concept effectuates an improvement in the functionality (responsiveness, proprioception and strength) along with an increase in exertion capacity (dosage exertion). Each is dependent on the other. By attaining sufficient muscular strength and balance, a functional improvement and therefore optimal spinal movement is possible.

This is achieved by way of the guided movements on the 1st –LBE and the support and corrections of the physical therapist. During spinal extension, the force of gravity is eliminated and thus the vertebrae are gently pulled apart, minimizing the pressure on the disks. The extension takes place at the muscular level. The muscles are "shown" how they should move. The physiological development of the movement into singular spinal segments enables the correction of disorders and misalignments.

This neurological steering greatly improves the geometry and movement of the vertebral segments with respect to one another and to the components within the vertebral segments, as well as their equilibrium. The end result is that the vertebrae return to their original positions and move optimally.

Every spine can be treated individually using a moderate, dosage modification of the range of motion (three-dimensional movement in flexion, extension, lateral flexion, and rotation), taking into consideration the type of dysfunction [13].

Furthermore, with the 1st –LBE, the muscles surrounding the spine attain a highly effective, intensively focused increase in strength. The effort intensity is determined for each patient individually.

Muscle strength capacity refers to the maximum level at which a muscle can perform a typical dynamic or static exertion in a specific time interval and intensity, without any overstrain. Specifically strengthening a patient's atrophied paravertebral muscle group also improves muscular balance.

According to the Dynasom therapy concept using 1st–LBE, the muscle is steered and activated for exertions specifically opposing/contrary to the misalignment to successfully work against it.

Muscle strength and balance, and spinal function are inter-dependent. Utilized together, they can bring about a structural change at the origin of the spinal dysfunction/ailment. Such changes can be seen on the x-rays of representative patients shown in Figures 12 and 13.

Activating the back muscles reduces the pressure on the spine joints and intervertebral discs, which increases the volume of the intervertebral discs and the slipping of vertebrae is reduced.

Functional scoliosis in different age groups, even among those with structural components, as well as structural scoliosis up to a certain age, can be partially corrected. This positively influences the entire statics and biomechanics of the spine, which guarantees the patient a long-term improvement in posture and movement.

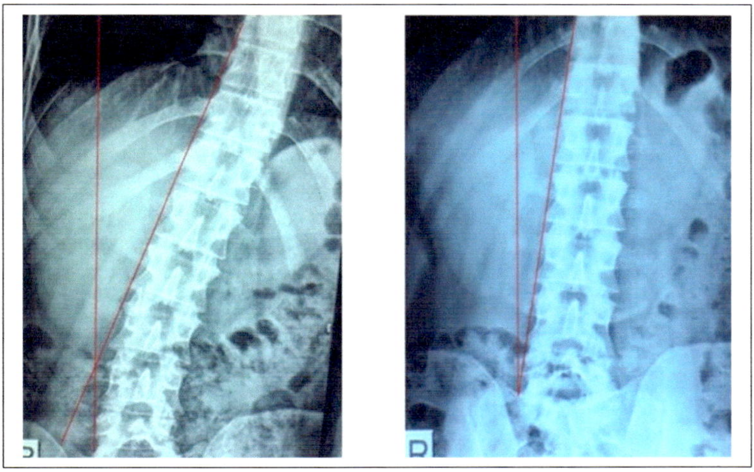

Figure 12: 12.1. Prior to treatment with 1st –LBE: left convex scoliosis of 23°, causing spinal disorder. 12.2. After 18 therapy sessions with 1st –LBE: scoliosis was corrected and reduced to 8°, and the LBP disappeared

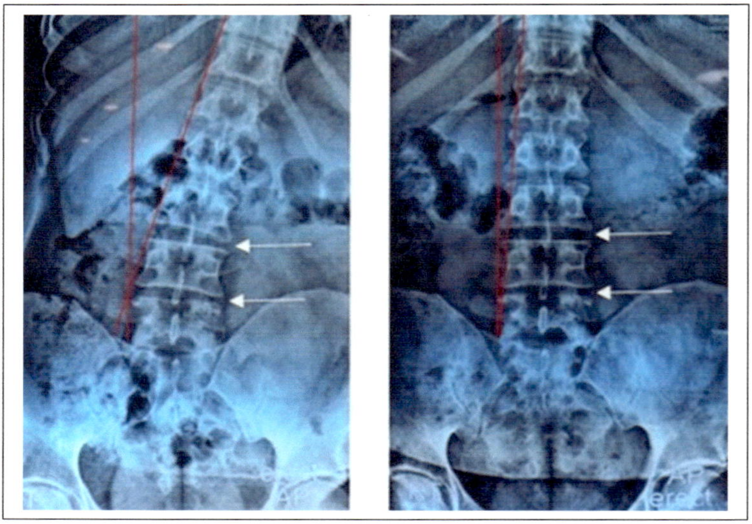

Figure 13: 13.1. Prior to treatment with 1st –LBE: left convex scoliosis of 19°, causing spinal disorder. 13.2. After 18 therapy sessions with 1st –LBE: the scoliosis was corrected to minimum. Therefore, the LBP disappeared

5.4.4. Treating LBP

How do we treat pain and find difference between the types of muscle fibers?

By regulating the muscle geometry. The function of every muscle fiber in a muscle is governed by this regulation. Both tension and strength are controlled, and the tensions of individual muscle fibers are coordinated with one another.

When the tension in a single muscle fiber is too high, the movement is disturbed, and pain occurs. As a result, other organs, including the lungs and heart are affected and also suffer. (These rules do not apply to exertion pain).

My controlled exertion therapy normalizes and harmonizes the tension in the muscle fibers independently of the patient's strength level through specific tension and relaxation.

The 1st–LBE apparatus defines which strength (exertion) level that should be selected. The muscles become stronger and the spine is re-stabilized. The goals of the therapy are two-fold: 1) the patient's average exertion level is defined; and 2) the patient's maximum level of exertion of his/her spine, without damaging the spine, is defined.

Exertion pain affects 10% of back patients, involving mostly fast-twitch fibers. This reflects a physiological pain reaction, occurring through muscle contractions and is, independent of the exertion level (anaerobic), and immediately disappears when the muscles stop contracting.

However, if the patient does not understand this normal physiological response this can lead to a pathological change. Consequently, the patient becomes very cautious, causing muscle weakness that can lead to other ailments, such as lumbar spine syndrome. Exertion pain involving only fast-twitch fibers that can be diagnosed and treated successfully with the 1st–LBE apparatus (Fig. 14).

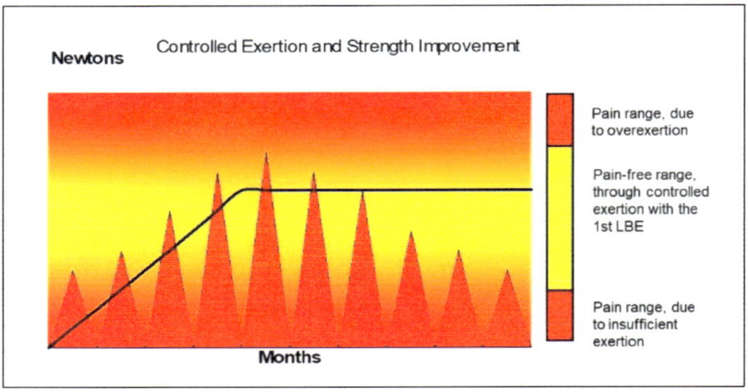

Fig. 14. Exertion pain increases due to anaerobic contractions in fast-twitch fibers. The red bars show increasing pain through the muscles during workout that disappear after a minute or two when the movement stops. 10% of back patients suffer from this physiological pain reaction, as clinically diagnosed by me using 1st–LBE and treated optimally.

5.4.5. Therapy treatment intensity using 1st–LBE

For back patients, two sessions a week for a total of 12–18 sessions on the 1st–LBE is sufficient to attain the desired stability, i.e. balance and toughness in the m. erector spinae system (Fig. 15).

This type of therapy intensity allows the muscles an optimal combination of exertion and regeneration, such that the unequal load distribution on other spinal components is reduced. Reducing overstrain makes possible the correction of functional scoliosis and spondylolisthesis, as well as the reestablishment of an optimal biomechanical function, to minimize the risk for lumbar vertebral syndrome in the future.

To maintain the achieved results, a maintenance program of one therapy session every 2 weeks for a total of nine therapy sessions in all [9]. Thus, the spine is protected from premature degenerative changes, and the risk of developing of further pathological change can be prevented.

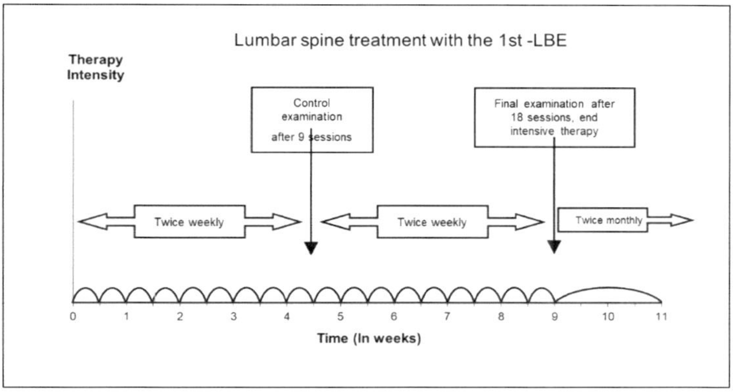

Fig. 15. Intensity of the Dynasom therapy using the 1st-LBE apparatus

Important Note:

At the end of each treatment series of nine therapy sessions, I assess whether further treatment is required. The precondition for continuation of treatment is a successful outcome of the completed series.

5.5. Cervical syndrome caused by lumbar spine dysfunction

Undoubtedly, the malfunction of the lower spine automatically causes an imbalance in the thoracic and cervical spine, which leads to a spinal disorder from cranial to sacral.

Undoubtedly, the malfunction of the lower spine automatically causes an imbalance in the thoracic and cervical spine, which leads to a spinal disorder from cranial to sacral.

This pain develops slowly and its character is clearly different from an accident complaint such as whiplash or a bacterial infection.

My diagnosis and therapy method is only performed if there is an additional problem with the cervical spine. This So it represents, a further form of lumbar spine treatment and is only initiated after the primary stabilization of the lumbar spine has already taken place, i.e. the fight against the causal problem has already begun.

The approach of my treatment of cervical spine is manual, consisting of flexion and extension, rotation L&R and lateral L&R movement performed using the hands and low resistance. A final massage to stimulate blood circulation can also be done for 5 minutes to encourage good muscle recovery (Fig. 16).

The patient's posture, restrictions on movement, and symptoms are addressed individually. During the massage, blood circulation is stimulated so that the muscles can recover well.

Based on the same principle as lumbar treatment, muscle function is improved and imbalances and tension are reduced. This has a positive influence on the position and movement of the cervical spine, which leads to a further reduction in pain in the area of the cervical spine.

These rules do not apply to cervical spine injuries such as those caused by accidents or inflammation due to bacterial infection.

Therefore, when diagnosing cervical spine complaints, we must take into account the malfunctions of the lumbar spine in order to achieve successful treatment of the cervical spine.

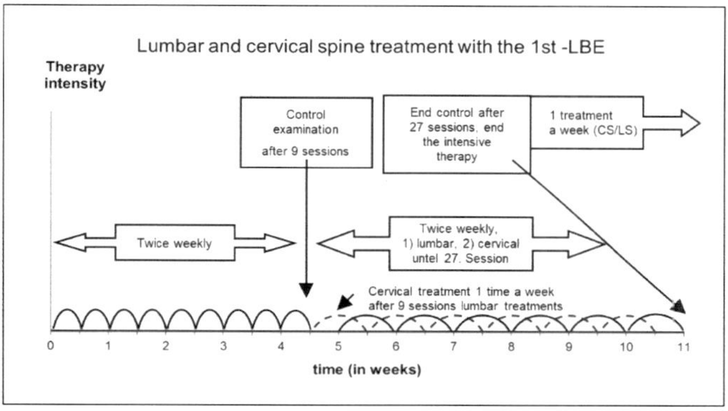

Fig. 16. Intensity of the treatment of the lumbar and cervical spine using 1st–LBE. I stabilized the lower back with 9 sessions; subsequently, I started treating the cervical spine, even if the patient has no LBP.

5.5.1. Frequency of lumbar syndromes

A lumbar syndrome is a set of signs and symptoms that are caused by functional disorders that lead to degenerative changes in the lumbar movement segments.

There are many risk factors for LBP: lack of education, poor physical and mental health, an unbalanced diet, lack of exercise, and an uncomfortable work environment [32]. Men are at risk of developing LBP; however, neck pain is more frequent among women. [33].

5.5.2. Age and gender distribution

Overall, men are slightly more affected by lumbar complaints than women [32], [33]. This predominance is not only due to an increased functional mechanical load, but also to an as yet unknown gender-specific factor.

In addition to its high frequency, the marked social significance of lumbar syndrome is that it mainly occurs in the middle of life (Fig. 17), affecting people at the peak of their performance. The symptoms are usually most frequent between ages 20–29 years, and continue to increase until the age of 60–65; subsequently, they slowly subside [32].

In this phase of life there is a special biomechanical constellation in the intervertebral discs: a still high level of swelling pressure of the gelatinous nucleus with already decreasing resistance of the annulus fibrosus, which raises the possibilities for the relocation of centrally located intervertebral disc tissue to the outside.

That means that the first signs of wear and tear start to have negative effects on the body. Fortunately, practicing the Dynasom concept, I can reduce, or perhaps even avoid, this development at an early stage. I cannot stop the wear and tear on the body; however, I can postpone it with less pain.

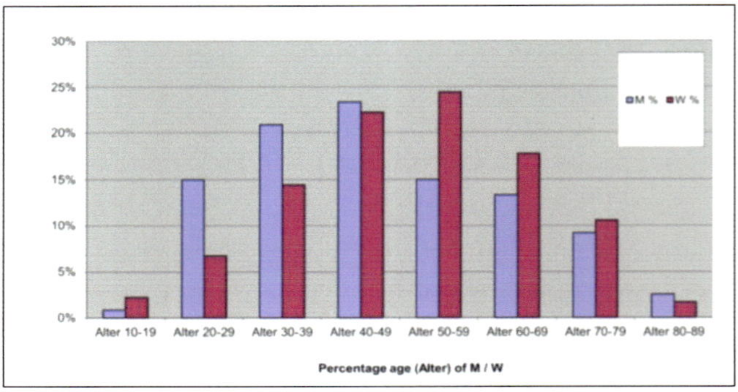

Fig. 17. The percentage of men and women patients in Switzerland and Germany. It can be observed that men are affected by LBP earlier in life than women; this is attributable to the difference in biological development.

5.5.3. Frequency of cervical syndromes

A cervical syndrome is marked by a symptom that is caused by dysfunction and degenerative changes in the cervical movement segments [34].

Frequency, age, and gender distribution: Some evidence suggests that responses to pain treatment may differ between women and men. Age also plays an important role in treatments, so I paid careful attention to age and gender during my diagnoses and therapy to avoid overloading [35].

Disc complaints in the cervical spine are very common, but not as common as in the lumbar spine. Women up to the age 50–60 are affected more often than men; after that, the men predominate. Acute clinical pictures affect more adolescents; chronic clinical pictures tend to affect older people. But the traumatic cervical syndrome occupies a special position. *"Both LBP and NP are common, with point and yearly prevalence (LBP/NP) around 18/14% and 38/26%, respectively".* [36].

5.6. Indications and contraindications

5.6.1. Indications for treatment of the spine.

a. Lumbar vertebral syndrome

b. Lumbar spondylolysis (pseudo-radicular) syndrome

c. Lumbar radicular syndrome

Etiology of these syndromes

a. Degenerative changes

b. Muscular insufficiency and imbalance

c. Misalignments and malformations

d. Postoperative conditions

e. Spondylolysis, spondylolisthesis

f. Spinal canal stenosis

g. Inflammations, rheumatic illnesses

h. Osteoporosis

The indications are independent of the age, gender, and profession of the patient.

5.6.2. Contraindications for treatment of the spine

Absolute contraindications

a. Sarcomas and metastases in the spine

b. Unconsolidated fractures

c. Cauda equina syndrome

d. Progressive neurological deficits with radicular syndromes

Relative contraindications

a. Acute radicular syndrome from the first few days up to the first few weeks

b. Advanced osteoporosis and osteomalacia

c. Inflammations, rheumatic illnesses in an acute, florid phase

5.7. Maintenance program for a healthy spine

After successful rehabilitation, the health of the spine in intimately related to the health of the body in general, and mainly depends on three basic elements:

A. Balanced nutrition. Anti-inflammatory and antioxidant foods, together with avoidance of alcohol, smoking, and sugar which all exacerbate body weight without benefit to prevent obesity, which can cause fatigue, lethargy, and disease.
B. Proper regular exercise. Forms of exercise that are enjoyable and also expend excess energy can help to expel bodily toxins and regulate the hormones of happiness, such as dopamine, serotonin, and endorphins.
C. Social connection. Communication with other members of the community can bring a sense of joyfulness and inspire spirit of cooperation and understanding. Such connections contribute to the formation of a supportive and cooperative society that understands the needs and interests of individuals to enjoy civilization and personal development.

5.7.1. Motion is the permanence of life

Movement is one secret of a healthy life, through which the circulatory system is activated to nourish the cells of the body with energy and vitality, and the disposal of waste. At the same time, movement plays an important role in the secretion of happiness hormones, which positively affect behavior, and the development of self-confidence.

Furthermore, it strengthens the muscles to more easily bear the weight of the body, which can save the joints, and reduce the risk of injury to the motor systems. With the help of balanced nutrition, movement activates the immune system of the human body, helping organs such as the heart, brain, liver, lungs, and kidneys to recover from fatigue and diseases of all kinds [37].

Here I clarify the benefits of regular exercise, which has the potential to improve human health. The movement has proved scientifically and practically to play a major role in our health!

This fact has become clear in all Details of human life and especially rid of diseases and works to increase the vitality. This in turn affects positively both physical and psychological development [2], [38].

Any muscle in the human body that is exercised regularly will consume the energy stored in the working muscle and form lactic acid (during strenuous exercise) as a waste. This activates the circulatory system in general, and the muscles to work especially hard to get rid of the lactic acid and replace it with new energy sources including resources such as oxygen and glucose.

This process activates the liver to send its energy stores to depleted muscles, thus renewing their vitality [39, 40].

5.7.2. Muscle workouts produce myokines

Scientists have found that muscle contractions produce hormone-like substances called myokines [41], [42]. This substance helps to burn stored energy, regulate the work of hormones, and activate the hormones of happiness, such as dopamine, serotonin, and endorphins, which increase the vitality.

These molecules are starting to be used against cancer cells and to overcome diabetes and gastrointestinal diseases [43]. That indicates that this substance has an optimal effect on the well-being of individuals and has a positive impact on physical and psychological conditions.

A high body weight or presence of disease can complicate the flow of blood circulation and play an important role in patients who have difficulty moving.

The result is compromised safety of body organs, and muscle weakness, which harm the joints, especially the spine.

Therefore, we must combat the lack of movement as part of our approach to disease treatment, providing our patients with a scientific basis for our health recommendations, which typically include regular exercise.

The most important elements of movement comprise the skills that begin from the first days of life, and continue to develop in accordance with the quantity and quality of exercise during childhood and beyond. Congenital and acquired diseases also play an important role in the capacity for activity, especially in the period of growth or adulthood.

Irrespective of growth, motor skills can be developed at any age provided there is communication of the required information and proper supervision to eliminate errors and avoid negative consequences, such as injury and misinterpretation.

There are also clear benefits of physical movement on our psychology that imply broad impacts on human health and behavior [44].

All scientific research on growth during childhood supports the notion that a healthy rate of growth is movement-dependent. Researchers recommend an outdoor activity to improve the health of children [45]. At the same time, nutrition plays a complementary role in muscle building, which is the real engine of the human body.

The movement works to activate the blood circulation and thus maintain metabolic activities and vitality of the body. It is customary to develop the muscles through organized and continuous movements, or through resistance movements that work to increase the capacity of muscle fibers.

Doing sports regularly helps to release the endorphin hormones, which are associated with a sense of happiness in humans [46].

Similarly, the muscles produce hormone-like substances called myokines, which play roles in burning carbohydrates and excess fat, and have been used in the treatment of diabetes, cancer, psychological diseases and digestive disorders.

The importance of exercise is unmistakable, and we must advise our populations to be physically active [47], [48].

My invention of the 1st –LBE, an anti-gravitational non-surgical, and non-pharmaceutical spinal care solution, has enabled me to develop my treatment concept Dynasom that includes the diagnosing of the main causes of back pain so that they may be overcome, thereby eliminating the pain using movement only without medication or surgical interventions. My patients have received joyful results [10].

Muscle contraction requires a certain level of heat, generated through the interactions of actin and myosin. These regulate the hormones of the body and activate the blood circulation, which in turn helps to restore the healing of cells after fatigue or disease. Movements also lead to the release of endorphins which increase one's sense of happiness and affect behavior positively.

Therefore, movement plays important roles in preventing and treating joint diseases, diabetes, cancer, digestive diseases, and mental illness.

In summary, mechanical movement and the chemical reactions induced by it improve the physical and psychological health of humans. The right kinds of movement strengthen the muscles and maintain the cohesion joints, enabling people to easily raise and move their body weight. For these reasons, the art of motion is at the forefront of other sciences in improving human health, overcoming fatigue and disease, and prolonging life.

Chapter six

6. Participants/Patients

From 4000 back patients at my rehabilitation centers 1) Stadelhofen, Zurich, Switzerland (2003–2010), 2) Wetzikon, Switzerland (2003–2010), and 3) Dynasom Academy Konstanz Germany (2011–2017), 4) Sporty Spine Baghdad/Iraq (2018–2019), I have evaluated 1,580 patients who met the following criteria:

1. First research population (already published): spinal instability, 440 patients

a. Aged 16–92 years (mean age, M = 48, F = 53 years)
b. Symptoms were present for an average of 8 months prior to treatment
c. Lower back pain
d. Radiating pain
e. Combination of LBP and radiating pain in one leg

The diagnoses of the patients were categorized as:

a. 153 patients with functional scoliosis
b. 28 patients with spondylolisthesis
c. 32 patients with herniated discs
d. 70 patients with degenerative diseases
e. 141 patients with multi-segmental degenerative changes
f. 16 patients without specific pathology

2. Second research population (already published): leg length discrepancy, 210 patients

a. Aged 18–65 years
b. The average duration of symptoms was 6 months
c. Leg length discrepancies of 3–9 mm

d. Lower back pain

The diagnosis of the patients was functional scoliosis, which caused by LLD.

3. Third research population (not published yet): spinal instability and leg length discrepancy, 930 patients

a. Ranging in age from 15 to 65 years
b. Symptoms were present for >12 weeks prior to treatment
c. Lower back pain
d. Combination of LBP and radiating pain in one leg

The diagnoses of the patients were categorized as:

a. Disc bulge
b. Intervertebral disc protrusion
c. Disc prolapse
d. Nerve roots compression
e. No facet syndrome
f. No spinal channel stenosis
g. No fractions

I examined my patients through 1st–LBE, requested the required X-ray scans and guided them to understand the primary causes of their problem.

My patients are treated by me or a well-trained physiotherapist using the 1st–LBE in the above-mentioned centers as follows:

A. All my patients **[1,580]** received physical therapy to improve the three-dimensional spinal function using 1st–LBE; 12–18 therapy sessions within 6–8 weeks, patients
with LLD were also given orthopedic heel cushions made of leather with a firm foam underside.

B. For research purposes and comparison: **50 patients** with spinal instability and LLD received physical therapy alone to improve three-dimensional spine function; 12 therapy sessions within 6 weeks.
C. I also evaluated 50 patients who received orthopedic heel cushions to adjust the leg length difference within 6 weeks without any additional program.

Physical therapy for all aforementioned groups was carried out by me and my trained physiotherapist (under my supervision) on the self-developed diagnostic and therapy device 1st –LBE. The main goal of this physical therapy was to improve three-dimensional spine function. The device allows an exact measurement of the load and balance of the m. erector spinae system (left or right, lateral or rotation, and flexion and extension, i.e. three-dimensional), measured in newton and degrees during inclination and reclination.

This device allows us to observe, analyze and correct the abnormalities of a movement. The patient's upper body mass was balanced on the device to biomechanically remove the effects of gravity on the spine and to integrate the necessary load and balance (correction) in the new movements.

After securing the balance in the erector spinae system between L&R in the first 3– 4 therapy sessions, an intensive targeted muscle building program was carried out to increase the resilience. Resistance was increased by 5% in each session until the goals (balance and toughness) were achieved: equivalent to 60% of body weight for male patients, and 50% of body weight for female patients.

Each therapy session lasted 20–30 min and included two therapy series. In each series there are 20–30 repetitions within 150 s (submaximal = anaerobic load) with a break of 1– 2 minutes between the series. The physical therapy was carried out twice a week for 6 weeks. Patients completed the pain questionnaire before therapy and after 6 weeks of therapy (12 sessions; conclusion of therapy). The follow-up pain questionnaire was not completed until 6–12 months after completion of therapy.

Important note:

All Patients were evaluated using the low back pain rating scale (LBPRS) [49], [50]. The language of the questionnaires was German and translated into English (Tables 1, 2, and fig. 18). For the duration of the therapy program, we did not allow patients to take any medication or participate in other activities or therapies.

Chapter seven

7. Results

Retrospective analysis of patient records (1,580 patients): I evaluated the three research groups: 1) spinal instability and LBP, 2) leg length discrepancy with LBP, and 3) LBP caused by spinal instability and LLD.

To evaluate the data, I divided the results into two groups and determined the percentage of patients found a significant reduction in LBP after physical therapy using 1st–LBE for 6–18 sessions.

Fifty patients with LBP and LLD received only orthopedic heel cushions; therefore, 22 patients had a worse result. Fifty participants with LBP and LLD received only physical therapy with 1st–LBE, 42 of them had a reduced LBP for only 1–2 days.

All other participants received physical therapy with 1st–LBE to improve the toughness and balance of the m. erector spinae twice a week for 9–18 sessions and compensate for LLD, if available.

A total of 1% of participants experienced increased LBP, 22% did not find any reduction in LBP, 3% experienced LBP reduction for 1–2 days only, and 74% had a significant decrease in LBP (Table 1).

Table 1. The three participant's groups of 1,580 patients and the percentage of response from patients with reduced and unreduced LBP after treatment with 1st–LBE for 6–18 sessions

Patients groups	LBP= worse	LBP= non reduced	LBP= 1-2 days reduced	**LBP= significant reduced**	Total
1st research group T1		56		84	140
1st research group T2		33		267	300
2nd research group T1	22	28			50
2nd research group T2		8	42		50
2nd research group T3		15		95	110
3rd research group T1		139		438	577
3rd research group T2		62		291	353
Total participants	22	341	42	**1175**	**1580**
percentage of total	1.00%	22.00%	3%	**74%**	**100%**

50 patients only received orthopedic heel cushions, so 22 patients had a worse result

50 participants had a LLD, but only received physical therapy with the 1st LBE, 42 of them had a reduced LBP for only 1-2 days

Patients aged 15 to 65 years: average age for men 45 years and for women 50 years

74% of patients reported a significant reduction of LBP after treating with the 1st -LBE, and compensating for the LLD (where it exists)

When evaluating 1,175 patients with a significant LBP reduction, a positive relationship was found between the increasing of the toughness with the balance of m. erector spinae and LBP relief by compensating for the LLD.

Some patients quickly achieved the optimal toughness and balance (equivalent to 60% and 50% of body weight for male and female patients, respectively) and others slowly. This helped them reduce the LBP or be free from back pain $r\ (9) = 0.98$, $p < 0.001$ (Table 2).

After eliminating the main causes of LBP, the pain subsided or disappeared in 74% of patients who followed instructions and completed the entire program (Tables 1, 2).

The high patient-satisfaction rates after completing the maintenance therapy program using 1st–LBE twice every month for 6–12 months revealed the constant success of being active. The good physical and mental states allowed the patients to avoid the LBP recurrence (Fig. 18).

Table 2: Comparison of LBP after completion of the whole program of 9–18 therapy sessions using the 1st LBE and the improvement of the toughness (tough_imp) of m. erector spinae in the percentage of patient weight (W&M for 1,175 patients).

Results of LBPRS	tough_imp/women	tough_imp/men	**Patients**	
6	50%	60%	411	
5	45%	55%	319	r (9)= 0.98
5	40%	50%	210	
4	35%	45%	129	**p < .001**
4	30%	40%	106	
3	25%	35%		**statically significant**
3	20%	30%		
2	15%	25%		
2	10%	20%		
1	5%	10%		
1	0%	5%		
			1175	

The percentage of toughness improvement (togh_imp) in the m. erector spinae in terms of body weight in W&M.

Results of LBPRS, 6=no more LBP, 5=much better, 4=better, 3=unchanged, 2=bad, 1=worse

Patients aged from 15 to 65 years: mean age for males, 45 years and for females, 50 years

There was a significant positive relationship between the increasing of the toughness with the balance of m. erector spinae and LBP relief by compensating for the LLD among the participants, r(9)= 98, p < .001

Here are more details:

1. First group: 6–9 therapy sessions (9% of the total patients).

A small number, **56** Patients (4%) of the entire patient population, which represented 40% of patients in the first group, experienced no improvement; thus no further therapy treatments were recommended for the following reasons:

a) 75% with advanced multi-segmental pain symptoms

b) 7% multi-morbid patients

c) 5% looking for a quick solution to their pain

d) 5% not interested in working actively

e) 3% traumatized

f) 3% depressive

g) 2% other factors

Another **84** patients (5%) of the entire patient population, represented 60% of patients in the first group, reported a significant reduction of LBP. However, these patients discontinued treatment for various other reasons:

a) 30% felt good and did not want to continue treatment
b) 20% had difficulties with traveling and time pressures due to work or personal situation
c) 20% had a third-party doctor who recommended discontinuation of treatment.
d) 15% had health insurance that did not cover therapy, and insurer recommended discontinuation of treatment.
e) 10% thought the therapy was too expensive
f) 5% other factors

2. Second group: 12–18 therapy sessions (91% of total patients).

Only **349** patients (22%) of the entire patient population (24% of the second patient group) experienced no change; therefore, a maintenance program was not recommended. However, **1091** patients (69%) of all patients (76% of the second patient group) reported a significant improvement and were recommended a maintenance program of 6– 9 therapy sessions twice monthly, with a further follow-up assessment after 6– 12 months.

Goals of the maintenance program:

1) Anchoring of the achieved therapy results.

2) Long-term maintenance of actual muscle strength and balance.

3) Further reduction of spinal symptoms where possible

Advantages of the maintenance program:

1) The patient becomes independent and learns how to deal with their pain (i.e. residual symptoms), as well as to take responsibility for their well-being.
2) The patient is monitored constantly in case there are any adversities, such as a deterioration of the condition caused by over-strain or wrong movement.
3) The maintenance program takes place over a longer time period, ensuring a long-term improvement of the symptoms.
4) Long-term observance of the symptoms in different circumstances is advantageous for the overall benefit of the patient.

Results of the follow-up questionnaire assessment 6–12 months after therapy: 457 of my patients from Switzerland and Germany registered for follow-up, here are the results.

About one-third (159 patients, 35%) of patients reported being pain-free and feeling that the therapy was the best that they had ever received. Nearly half (206 patients, 45%) reported being very satisfied and confirmed that the therapy results were providing a long-term benefit; they assessed the therapy as "good". A total of 92 patients (20%) reported being satisfied, but that it was not better than other therapy alternatives (Fig. 18).

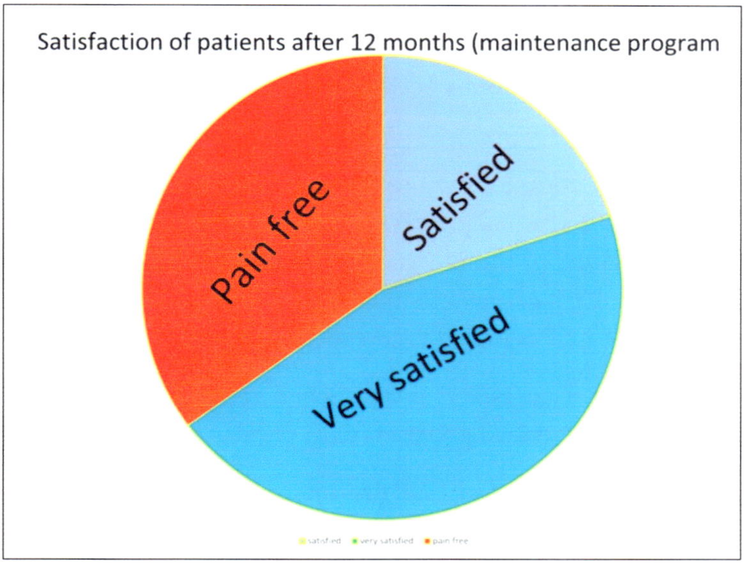

Fig. 18. Results of the aftercare satisfaction after maintenance program therapy with 1st-LEB twice a month for 6–12 months for 457 patients by compensating for the existing LLD

Summary of key results:

LBP can be eliminated by improving the three-dimensional function of the spine with the 1st–LBE. This gives the m. erector spinae toughness and balance. Furthermore, compensating for the LLD (if available) plays a key role in success. Maintaining the therapy success could be ensured by a regular training program; this avoids recruiting LBP.

Many health problems during the old age can be avoided by identifying the primary LBP causes and treating them optimally after the growth phase.

Diagnosing the main causes of LBP, such as weakness and imbalance of the m. erector spinae using 1st–LBE and LLD using the X-ray hips-pelvis standing offers a good chance to eliminate LBP using targeted active therapy.

The therapy course aimed to improve the three-dimensional function of the spine gradually with the 1st–LBE by optimizing the toughness and balance of the m. erector spinae and compensation of the LLD (if available). This achievement supports 70%–80% of back patients in the treatment of LBP without medication and surgery.

To maintain success and avoid recurrence of LBP, patients have to go through a maintenance program with regular exercise.

If these main causes of LBP are found after the growth phase and eliminated at an early stage, back pain can be avoided.

Discussion:

many patients who consulted me were shocked and demoralized by the diagnoses of clinicians. Certain patients are scared of overdoing medication and surgery because certain medications and operations damage the nerves and muscles and make rehabilitation more difficult. It was too difficult to succeed with such patients.

Therefore, I completed the success of my entire therapy with Dynasom concept, using the 1st-LBE due to the improvement of the toughness and the balance of the m. erector spinae dependent. In other words, these muscles play a major role in eliminating the LBP after compensating for the LLD.

If the muscles fail, there is no success. This happens with muscle diseases, nerve diseases, injuries, mental illnesses, fractures, nerve damage due to other diseases such as diabetes mellitus, heart and blood diseases. In such cases, the patients have to be treated differently.

80% of individuals have good m. erector spinae that can ensure a healthy spine. These are a good potential to relieve LBP.

Success of the treatment also depends on lifestyle and habits. Patients should understand the spinal problems better and exercise regularly to gain joy, control a balanced diet with pleasure, and maintain positive communication with society.

In conclusion, clinicians should identify the main causes of LBP after the growth phase, such as weakness and imbalance of the m. erector spinae and LLD. These measurements should also be taken from the age of 18 to avoid back pain as much as possible in life.

Therapists should also specialize in treating spinal diseases and educate themselves on treatment of the back pain. As a result, patients are better informed and treated.

Finally, the patients should take minimal medication and only undergo spinal surgery in extreme cases.

Chapter eight

8. Discussion

Undiscovered primary causes of LBP in conventional medicine:

The results of my study refute those of other comparable studies, which tolerated a LLD of up to 10 mm without therapeutic consequence [51,52]. A LLD between 3– 9 mm can cause considerable damage to the spine. Compensating for LLD using only orthopedic heel cushions is insufficient to optimally eliminate the back pain.

Conventional medical literature has discussed spinal instability for > 50 years, but has never given a precise description of the functional problems that arise outside of a specific disease qualification. As an example, minimal scoliosis of < 10°, and minimal spondylolisthesis (Anterolisthesis or Retrolisthesis) of 3– 5 mm have never taken seriously. Likewise, a LLD of < 10 mm is not accounted for, nor is an imbalance between the L&R in the m. erector spinae system ever discussed.

After > 20 years of practical experience in this field, which led me to define the instability of the spine, I have proven that it plays a major role in the spinal disorders that cause LBP [10].

The LLD and the weakness of the m. erector spinae with an imbalance between the L&R sides are the main causes of spinal instability, which leads directly or indirectly to LBP [11].

Therefore, practitioners should check these three important causes of LBP seriously, and place high value on the diagnosis and treatment of LBP [53].

The side effects of pharmaceutical medications can cause damage to the musculoskeletal system that outweighs any benefits of soothing the LBP. It has become apparent in recent years that many patients became addicted to affective but strong opioids that led to many secondary damages in bodily organs as a result of long-term use or abuse. "Adverse effects of opioid administration include sedation, dizziness, nausea, vomiting, constipation, dependency and tolerance, and respiratory depression. The most common adverse effect of opioid use is constipation" [54].

Herniated disc operations, in which the intervertebral discs are partially removed, result in new problems due to the reduction in height (e.g. facet joint syndrome). Intervertebral disc prosthesis operations that artificially replace the intervertebral discs have not yet passed the test of time, and in any case do not resolve the cause of the problem "Globally the method is declining and in many health care financing models it is not an approved treatment" [55].

Spinal fusion operations, which block one or more movement segments, eliminate the function of the intervertebral discs in the affected movement segments. Other, movement segments are stressed as a result, creating a risk of a screw breakage and disruptions at the transition to the movable segments. The screws used in the fusion surgery also replace the muscle function in the spine, which is why the muscles atrophy a few years later.

Prof. Dr. Andre Busato has described the frequent spinal operations in Switzerland through the use of medical services from the health insurance company as a financial interest not supported by medical necessity [56].

For these reasons, I do not consider medication or surgery separately as an optimal solution to treat back pain. Rather, I consider the negative effects of the drugs and the limiting effects of spinal operations on the movement of the spine, as well as the damage to the nerves and muscles surrounding it, to be of harm to human activity and vitality, and to society as a whole. In my opinion, medication and spinal surgeries only treat the symptoms, and overstep the main causes.

My method, has been proven both scientifically and practically to relieve LBP in 70– 80 % of patients who had not already found a solution to their problem [10], [11]. It also helps to revitalize the vertebral column to its previous level or better. With this work, I have created a convincing alternative to spine surgery, giving patients a way to avoid pain medications with the risk of abuse and instead pursue a healthy, enjoyable life.

A common problem with joint surgeries, especially those of the ankle, knee, or hip joints is the variety of pain sources in the affected joint. Because the large joints act constantly to perform all the required bodily movements, they can be a possible source of pain. Because the spine is viewed as an axis of motion, it contributes to joint pain in a certain percentage (this rule does not apply to rheumatoid arthritis).

Clarification through practical experience: my Swiss surgeon college Dr. Arnold Rueegg Wetzikon-CH told me at the end of 2003 that one of his patients continues to suffer from 30% of hip pain after a joint replacement surgery. He believed that the pain in the hip joint originates in the spine.

However, the patient did not suffer from back pain; therefore, the spine was ruled out as the source of pain. The patient was aware of their health and allowed us to investigate this case.

I found a LLD, which in turn led to a minimal functional scoliosis; accordingly, I treated the lower back with ideal results using my Dynasom concept and the 1st–LBE and equation the LLD. The 30% of pain in the hip disappeared after 9 therapy sessions. Subsequently, we (Dr. Arnold Rueegg and I) learned that the source of the pain was the spinal instability, which was caused by LLD. We learned a lot from this lesson and Dr. Arnold Rueegg used the experience gained in his treatments and improved his surgical concept. He achieved better results in the surgical treatment of the knee and hips. After many successful cases, we recognized the benefit of this treatment and the experience evolved into a base concept that can be applied before and after joint surgery.

Through this experience, we found that LLD affected the body by causing pain in the joints, including in the spine, and how can we treat these origins of pain. On this basis, we published our research in 2016.

That is why I recommend that joint surgeons should research these findings to make the experience useful and beneficial or to implement this new knowledge on a scientific and practical level.

Furthermore, the Dynasom rehabilitations concept should be implemented in any spinal surgical department as a pre- and postoperative practice to provide better results in each stage of joint and spinal treatment. Working together is an optimal way to gain success.

The progress of my Dynasom concept, fits exactly with the number 3 of the 17 UNESCO 2030 goals: better health and well-being. While success with my treatment concept depends on the stage of the patient's spinal problem, the patient's level of background knowledge and enthusiasm for recovery play equally important roles.

The discussion of the results:

Lower back pain (LBP) is mechanical in nature and is the most common health issue worldwide, especially in developed countries. The loss of jobs and early retirement are part of the stress and disappointment with losing quality of life and prosperity.

LBP restricts movement and causes a lack of self-confidence and malaise. When these are developed among individuals, it has a negative impact on society.

Conventional medicine does not focus on the main causes of LBP and focuses on treating symptoms. That is why 60%–80% of adults worldwide suffer from LBP.

It starts with the family doctor, who does not have enough time for back patients. He quickly prescribes medication to relieve the pain or refers the patient to a physiotherapist, who only deals with the problem in general, without specialty.

The patient realizes that the medication is only a sedative and has a side effects or that the physiotherapist is overstrained with the back problem.

Thus, the first misdiagnosis is performed by the family doctor, which triggers the initial negative reaction of the patient. The next is the management of pain therapy (infiltration), which can only work for a limited period of time to keep the pain under control. If this does not work, the patient begins to look for alternative treatments or consider surgery without calculating the consequences.

The pain burdens the patient and the pressure in professional and private lives increases. As a result, the patient feels alone to counteract the problem. This can trigger a psychological problem, causing the patient to become disoriented.

I have broken this vicious cycle with the patients with a therapy that deals with the main causes of LBP without medication or surgery.

These causes of LBP were previously unknown, and I achieved these results in my special centers (Switzerland, Germany, and Iraq) that deal primarily with LBP under principles of movement science (treatment) as a physical active therapy.

The search for the major causes of LBP was my goal. Through my invention of the 1st–LBE (anti-gravitation system) I examined and evaluated my patients and found the following:

1) **99% have spinal instability, caused by weakness and imbalance in m. erector spinae between L&R**

2) **95% have deficit in strength and range of motion in m. erector spinae that causes LBP**
3) **70% have LLD of 3–9 mm that causes spinal instability, causing LBP**
4) **10% have fast-twtich fibers in m. erector spinae, which causes physiological LBP**

I achieved my precise diagnosis using the following material:

a) My self-developed 1st–LBE (anti-gravitation system), a device that measures every Newton and every degree of three-dimensional movements of the spine.
b) The X-rays standing (lumbosacral spine a.p./lat.) to document the abnormality in the lumbar spine.
c) The standing X-ray (hips-pelvis with a.p.) to determine the LLD of 3–9 mm and document anomalies, especially in sacroiliac joints.

With my active therapy, I improved the toughness (equivalent to 60% of body weight of male and 50% of body weight of female patients) and balance (between L&R) of the m. erector spine with using 1st–LBE apparatus). In addition, I compensated for the LLD (where it exists) using orthopedic heel cushions.

Moreover, I found and improved the optimal range of motion between flexion and extension for patients with LBP to 45°–51° flexion and a 9°–6° extension; this was enough to ensure necessary spinal function for daily requirements.

Therefore, the patients had sufficient strength to correct the imbalance between L&R, this ensures the three-dimensional function of the spine, which serves as protection to the spinal elements, and eliminates the major causes of LBP in 9–12 sessions.

I also diagnosed 10% of patients with their physiological LBP (exertion pain), which is due to contractions of the fast twitch fibers in m. erector spinae. The patients needed 3–5 therapy sessions to descry these kind of fibers; subsequently, I set up a suitable program and treated them optimally.

With this study, I achieved the following results with patients who followed my instructions

1. **74% were satisfied with the therapy effect after 9–12 Therapy sessions:**
   a) 24% no longer had LBP after three therapy sessions,
   b) 40% were very satisfied with the reduction of their LBP,
   c) 10% have residual LBP; however, they were satisfied with the therapy, but they wished further improvement.

2. **26% were not satisfied with the result of the Therapy effect for various reasons:**
   a) They have already advanced spinal damage (multi-segmental),
   b) Pre-existing diseases
   c) Others

Conclusions:

In total, 80% of the population have a good quality of m. erector spinae, and can work perfectly to eliminate LBP without medications and spinal surgery, but the patients do not know about this. It is my duty to present these achievements to expert groups and society to work with back muscles and eliminate LBP. This can contribute to a healthy life.

Twice a week is the best therapy frequency to improve the m. erector spinae with the 1st–LBE. To maintain success, the patients should undergo a maintenance therapy program twice a month and exercise regularly for 20–30 minutes a day and at least five times a week.

I trained 10 physiotherapists in my rehabilitation centers on the knowledge and my practical experience, so they improved their knowledge in the radiology, muscle and nerve physiology, and biomechanics of the spine.

Therefore, they were able to implement my therapy using 1st–LBE and treat my patients successfully. Accordingly, I have developed an education program to make the knowledge understandable for physicians and therapists so they can benefit from this finding in their workplaces. 8 of 10 physiotherapists have learned to use my therapy method with the 1st–LBE as an employee in my rehabilitation centers and have performed well with the back patients.

Based on these results, I developed a further education program (theory and practice) over 3–6 months. In this program, Therapists will improve their knowledge of radiology, biomechanics and muscle-nerve physiology of the spine.

This achievement allowed a physiotherapist to practice the specialty of the spine in his workplace. Therefore, any physiotherapists have the opportunity to be specialized in the treatment of back patients, after completing the educational program because the spine is unique.

Chapter nine

9. General conclusions

Spinal instability is the major cause of spinal dysfunction, which leads to LBP. The three main causes of spinal instability are leg length discrepancy, weakness, and dysbalance of the m. erector spinae; therefore, each should be diagnosed and treated optimally and as soon as possible.

With a movement on the 1st–LBE, I can improve three-dimensional function of the spinal column and simultaneously optimize the performance of the m. erector spinae, by means of various resistances in stages (dosage exertion).

Despite the fact that I work with anaerobic performance, I should also perform therapy with the erector spinae muscle at submaximal intensity, and not maximum intensity, to avoid overload, and still be able to relieve LBP.

Knowing each patient's type of muscle fibers and the right ways to improve their toughness, will contribute directly to providing adequate protection for the spine, and thus ensuring that nerves are protected from damage.

Discovering a difference in leg length after the age of 17 helps patients to effectively avoid building muscle with unbalanced motion and to reduce the occurrence of LBP.

By eliminating lumbar spine pain, 60% of neck pain disappears automatically.

Freeing the human body from LBP through movement contributes to the development of human health and happiness. It also plays an important role in the wealth of the individual and society.

LBP has a mechanical character, and is a global problem, therefore it can be diagnosed and treated optimally without medication (as needed) or spine surgeries (as necessary).

Attention to general health is essential for keeping the spine healthy, and can best be achieved through regular exercise performed correctly, balanced nutrition, and positive social communication.

A healthy life brings a healthy spine and contributes to a happy and healthy society.

Chapter ten

10. References

[1] John W Frymoyer. Back pain and sciatica. New England Journal of Medicine, 318(5):291–300, 1988.

[2] Peter J Carek, Sarah E Laibstain, and Stephen M Carek. Exercise for the treatment of depression and anxiety. The International Journal of Psychiatry in Medicine, 41(1):15–28, 2011.

[3] Scott A Paluska and Thomas L Schwenk. Physical activity and mental health. *Sports medicine*, 29(3):167–180, 2000.

[4] Simon Rosenbaum, Anne Tiedemann, Robert Stanton, Alexandra Parker, Anna Waterreus, Jackie Curtis, and Philip B Ward. Implementing evidence-based physical activity interventions for people with mental illness: an australian perspective. *Australasian Psychiatry*, 24(1):49–54, 2016.

[5] Pellis´e F Cedraschi C. Balagu´e F, Mannion AF. Non-specific low back pain. Lancet (London, England), 2012.

[6] Bin Wang and Peng Zhao. Worldwide research productivity in the field of back pain: A bibliometric analysis. *Medicine*, 97(40), 2018.

[7] Mohammad Reza Nourbakhsh and Amir Massoud Arab. Relationship between mechanical factors and incidence of low back pain. Journal of Orthopaedic & Sports Physical Therapy, 32(9):447–460, 2002.

[8] Robert Needham, Nachiappan Chockalingam, D Dunning, A Healy, EB Ahmed, and A Ward. The effect of leg length discrepancy on pelvis and spine kinematics during gait. Stud Health Technol Inform, 176:104–7, 2012.

[9] Moreno D'Amico, Piero Roncoletta, Francesca Di Felice, Daniele Porto, Rosagrazia Bellomo, and Raoul Saggini. Lbp and lower limb discrepancy: 3d evaluation of postural rebalancing via

underfoot wedge correction. Studies in health technology and informatics, 176:108—112, 2012.

[10]Adnan Mizher, A Rueegg, P Walthard, and T Hasler. Spinal instability. Manuelle Medizin, 50(3):211, 2012.

[11]A Mizher and A Rueegg. Considerable damage to the spine caused by small leg length discrepancy. MANUELLE MEDIZIN, 54(3):150–155, 2016.

[12]Rannisto S. Uitti J. Leg-length discrepancy is associated with low back pain among those who must stand while working. BMC Musculoskelet Disord., 2015.

[13]Jan W Raczkowski, Barbara Daniszewska, and Krystian Zolynski. Functional scoliosis caused by leg length discrepancy. Archives of medical science: AMS, 6(3):393, 2010.

[14]Anne F Mannion. Fibre type characteristics and function of the human paraspinal muscles: normal values and changes in association with low back pain. Journal of electromyography and kinesiology, 9(6):363–377, 1999.

[15]BEC Nienhaus and FA van de Laar. Lower back pain: understanding it is more important than treating it. Nederlands Tijdschrift Voor Geneeskunde, 161:D2032–D2032, 2017.

[16]Hollmann W. Basic physical activity, training and preventive medicine. Sports medicine, 2009.

[17]World Health Organization et al. WHO global recommendations on physical activity for health. geneva: World health organization; 2011.

[18]Sofi Sonesson, Joanna Kvist, Clare Ardern, Annika Osterberg, and Karin Gr¨avare Silbernagel.¨ Psychological factors are important to return to pre-injury sport activity after anterior cruciate ligament reconstruction: expect and motivate to satisfy. Knee surgery, sports traumatology, arthroscopy, 25(5):1375–1384, 2017.

[19]Joseph V Pergolizzi and Jo Ann LeQuang. Rehabilitation for low back pain: A narrative review for managing pain and improving

function in acute and chronic conditions. Pain and Therapy, pages 1–14, 2020.

[20]Maureen C Jensen, Michael N Brant-Zawadzki, Nancy Obuchowski, Michael T Modic, Dennis Malkasian, and Jeffrey S Ross. Magnetic resonance imaging of the lumbar spine in people without back pain. New England Journal of Medicine, 331(2):69–73, 1994.

[21]Shari Diamond and David Borenstein. Chronic low back pain in a working-age adult. Best practice & research Clinical rheumatology, 20(4):707–720, 2006.

[22]Johan WS Vlaeyen, Chris G Maher, Katja Wiech, Jan Van Zundert, Carolina Beraldo Meloto, Luda Diatchenko, Michele C Batti´e, Marielle Goossens, Bart Koes, and Steven J Linton. Low back pain (primer). Nature Reviews: Disease Primers, 2018.

[23]Julie A Hides, Gwendolen A Jull, and Carolyn A Richardson. Long-term effects of specific stabilizing exercises for first-episode low back pain. Spine, 26(11):e243–e248, 2001.

[24]M Shaughnessy and B Caulfield. A pilot study to investigate the effect of lumbar stabilisation exercise training on functional ability and quality of life in patients with chronic low back pain. International journal of rehabilitation research, 27(4):297–301, 2004.

[25]E Rasmussen-Barr, L Nilsson-Wikmar, and I Arvidsson. Stabilizing training compared with manual treatment in sub-acute and chronic low-back pain. Manual therapy, 8(4):233–241, 2003.

[26]Lucas Lima Ferreira, Regiane Rocha Costalonga, and Vitor Engr´acia Valenti. Therapy with physical exercises for low back pain. Revista Dor, 14(4):307–310, 2013.

[27]Lorimer Moseley. Combined physiotherapy and education is efficacious for chronic low back pain. Australian journal of physiotherapy, 48(4):297–302, 2002.

[28]Leena Niemist¨o, Tiina Lahtinen-Suopanki, Pekka Rissanen, Karl-August Lindgren, Seppo Sarna, and Heikki Hurri. A randomized trial of combined manipulation, stabilizing exercises, and physician consultation compared to physician consultation alone for chronic low back pain. Spine, 28(19):2185–2191, 2003.

[29]James Steele, Stewart Bruce-Low, and Dave Smith. A review of the clinical value of isolated lumbar extension resistance training for chronic low back pain. PM&R, 7(2):169–187, 2015.

[30]Vesa Lehtola, Hannu Luomajoki, Ville Leinonen, Sean Gibbons, and Olavi Airaksinen. Subclassification based specific movement control exercises are superior to general exercise in subacute low back pain when both are combined with manual therapy: A randomized controlled trial. BMC musculoskeletal disorders, 17(1):135, 2016.

[31]Bruno T Saragiotto, Christopher G Maher, Ti^e P Yamato, Leonardo OP Costa, Luciola C Menezes Costa, Raymond WJG Ostelo, and Luciana G Macedo. Motor control exercise for chronic non-specific low-back pain. Cochrane Database of Systematic Reviews, (1), 2016.

[32]Damian Hoy, Paul Brooks, Fiona Blyth, and Rachelle Buchbinder. The epidemiology of low back pain. Best practice & research Clinical rheumatology, 24(6):769–781, 2010.

[33]Eva Skillgate, Oscar Javier Pico-Espinosa, Johan Hallqvist, Tony Bohman, and Lena W Holm. Healthy lifestyle behavior and risk of long duration troublesome neck pain or low back pain among men and women: results from the stockholm public health cohort. Clinical epidemiology, 9:491, 2017.

[34]DG Hoy, M Protani, R De, and Rachelle Buchbinder. The epidemiology of neck pain. Best Practice & Research Clinical Rheumatology, 24(6):783–792, 2010.

[35]Roger B Fillingim, Christopher D King, Margarete C Ribeiro-Dasilva, Bridgett Rahim Williams, and Joseph L Riley III. Sex,

gender, and pain: a review of recent clinical and experimental findings. The journal of pain, 10(5):447–485, 2009.

[36]Rebecca J Crawford, Thomas Volken, Ren´e Schaffert, and Thomas Bucher. Higher low back and neck pain in final year swiss health professions' students: worrying susceptibilities identified in a multicenter comparison to the national population. BMC public health, 18(1):1188, 2018.

[37]Oliver C Witard and Derek Ball. The interaction between nutrition and exercise for promoting health and performance. The Proceedings of the Nutrition Society, 77(1):1—3, February 2018.

[38]Tongjian You, Nicole C Arsenis, Beth L Disanzo, and Michael J LaMonte. Effects of exercise training on chronic inflammation in obesity. Sports Medicine, 43(4):243–256, 2013.

[39]Michitaka Kato, Akira Kubo, Fumi Nihei, Michio Ogano, and Hisato Takagi. Effects of exercise training on exercise capacity, cardiac function, bmi, and quality of life in patients with atrial fibrillation: a meta-analysis of randomized-controlled trials. International Journal of Rehabilitation Research, 40(3):193–201, 2017.

[40]DDFM Rocco, LS Okuda, RS Pinto, FD Ferreira, SK Kubo, ER Nakandakare, ECR Quint˜ao, S Catanozi, and M Passarelli. Aerobic exercise improves reverse cholesterol transport in cholesteryl ester transfer protein transgenic mice. Lipids, 46(7):617–625, 2011.

[41]Pedersen BK, Steensberg A, Fischer C, Keller C, Keller P, Plomgaard P, Wolsk-Petersen E, Febbraio M. The metabolic role of IL-6 produced during exercise: is IL-6 an exercise factor? Proc Nutr Soc. 2004;63(2):263-7.

[42]K Ostrowski, T Rohde, M Zacho, S Asp, and BK Pedersen. Evidence that il-6 is produced in skeletal muscle during intense long-term muscle activity. J Physiol (Lond), 508:949–953, 1998.

[43]Pedersen BK[1], Fischer CP. Beneficial health effects of exercise--the role of IL-6 as a myokine. Trends Pharmacol Sci. 2007;28(4):152-6.

[44]Anita Slomski. Exercise delivers brain benefits. *Jama*, 321(12):1149–1149, 2019.

[45]Leyla E McCurdy, Kate E Winterbottom, Suril S Mehta, and James R Roberts. Using nature and outdoor activity to improve children's health. *Current problems in pediatric and adolescent health care*, 40(5):102–117, 2010.

[46]Mikkelsen K, Stojanovska L, Polenakovic M, Bosevski M, Apostolopoulos V. Exercise and mental health. Maturitas. 2017;106:48-56.

[47]Tero Pasanen, Samppa Tolvanen, Ari Heinonen, and Urho M Kujala. Exercise therapy for functional capacity in chronic diseases: an overview of meta-analyses of randomised controlled trials. British journal of sports medicine, 51(20):1459–1465, 2017.

[48]Prue Cormie, Eva M Zopf, Xiaochen Zhang, and Kathryn H Schmitz. The impact of exercise on cancer mortality, recurrence, and treatment-related adverse effects. *Epidemiologic reviews*, 39(1):71–92, 2017.

[49]Claus Manniche, Karsten Asmussen, Birgitte Lauritsen, Henrik Vinterberg, Svend Kreiner, and Alan Jordan. Low back pain rating scale: validation of a tool for assessment of low back pain. *Pain*, 57(3):317–326, 1994.

[50]http://www.orthoadc.com/files/2018/04/Spine-Follow-Up-Forms.pdf

[51]Hannes Manner. Malpositions and leg length differences in childhood and adolescence / Schulthess Klinik, Zurich.

[52]Gulbahge, Esma. Comparative study on the determination of leg length differences using sonographic and radiological methods presented. 2011, University of Munster.

[53]Peter R Croft, Gary J Macfarlane, Ann C Papageorgiou, Elaine Thomas, and Alan J Silman. Outcome of low back pain in general practice: a prospective study. *Bmj*, 316(7141):1356, 1998.

[54]Mahmoud Reza Khansari, Masour Reza Sohrabi, and Farhad Zamani. The useage of opioids and their adverse effects in gastrointestinal practice: a review. Middle East journal of digestive diseases, 5(1):5, 2013.

[55]Peter F¨orsth, Paul Gerdhem, and Olle Svensson. Lumbar disc prosthesis, a high risk treatment for low back pain. Lakartidningen, 117, 2020.

[56]Busato A. National Research Program "Musculoskeletal Health - Chronic Pain (NRP 53) 2014. MEM Research Center for Orthopedic Surgery, Institute for Evaluative Research in Orthopedic Surgery, University of Bern.

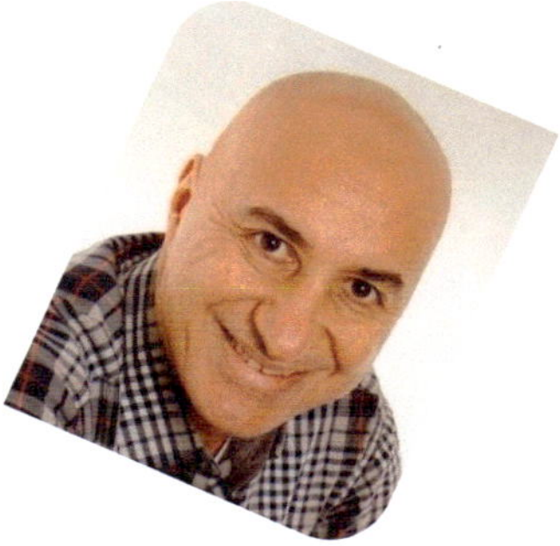

This doctoral thesis in health sciences by Atlantic International University of Dr. Adnan Mizher Samarmad presents his experiences from the last 20 years in the field of LBP, as a medical scientist aiming to investigate the main causes of LBP that have not yet been discovered!

In addition, the study includes the relationship between the cause and occurrence of LBP and a new method of overcoming painful symptoms naturally through exercise on the 1st -LBE with dosage exertion therapy without medication or surgery.

SportySpine.com

Made in United States
Cleveland, OH
05 November 2026

47646341R00059